HERE'S WHAT REVIEWERS HAD TO SAY ABOUT
FITNESS BEYOND 50: TURN BACK THE CLOCK

"At last, a REALLY helpful, easy-to-use guide to a healthy lifestyle for those of us past the 'middle years.' It provides motivation, education and behaviors to enhance lifestyle changes in a fun and very engaging format. I couldn't put it down!"

— Caroline Nielsen, Ph.D., Former Chair and Emeritus Professor, Graduate Program in Allied Health, University of Connecticut, Storrs, CT

"Harry, I really like this book project of yours! I'm a bit of a fitness and exercise freak, as you know. Yet in reading some of your materials and in the conversations they prompted, I've learned quite a bit. At the same time, the tone of the writing and the level at which you present things are quite engaging. You'll have the reader hooked before he or she knows it!"

— Theodore L. Brown, Ph.D., Emeritus Professor of Chemistry, University of Illinois, Urbana-Champaign, senior author of the best-selling text, *Chemistry: The Central Science*

"I wanted to thank you for the opportunity to read your chapter on exercise and the brain. I thought that it was informative and entertaining — with a good mix of both science and anecdote. I look forward to reading your book when it is published."

— Art Kramer, PH.D., Director of the Beckman Institute, University of Illinois, Urbana-Champaign

"Exercise really is the 'wonder-drug' that can treat diabetes, hypertension, osteoporosis, elevated cholesterol and many other age-related illnesses. You've given us the prescription, the only question is whether we will take our medicine.

"I really liked the 'Exercise and the Brain' chapter. Enough anecdotes to get information across, which was well done. Overall, this is the best chapter written so far. If anyone can read this chapter and not want to get out, they're crazy. Did I tell you I've started riding the towpath?

"I've been doing spin classes this winter. You've convinced me and I'm just proofing the book!"

— Chris M. Aland, M.D., Orthopedic and Sports Medicine, Langhorne, PA

"There's as much time after fifty as before and you want this time to be healthy, productive and fun. Harry offers advice, motivation and inspirational stories of real people on how to stay fit and young despite the passing years. Share this with those you love, it will positively change their lives!"

— Patricia Hedley, Managing Director,
General Atlantic, Greenwich, CT, a global growth investor

"Harry, thanks for the advance copy of your book. I'm loving it.

"I just turned fifty-five on Sunday. I've been a gym rat since about ninth grade, so you're truly preaching to the choir. Your book has reenergized me. I'm now focusing on the interval training aspect that you espouse. I've also started to log my workouts. Both of these measures are providing additional motivation for me. I work on taking one or two days a week off. If, for some unforeseen reason, I can't get my anticipated workout in, my skin feels like it wants to crawl off of my body. I guess I'm truly hooked. Your opus has helped me 'keep it fresh.' I don't know if this will all lead to a longer life, but I'm certain that it's leading me to a happier one."

— Russ Campion, Investment Banker, William Blair & Company, Chicago, IL

"I just finished the first seven chapters and must say it makes one think. You have a lot of very useful information in it and the individual stories are really great because they have more impact than a 'thou should.'

"It's a good book that I'm sure will be wonderful when you've got it all together. Based on what I've read, it would be one I'd recommend to everyone; and frankly, it would benefit younger folk. While there is a general increase in 'fitness,' there's nothing I'm aware of that is as specific or as broadly relevant as what you're creating."

— David Walls, Retired International Investment Banker, Santa Barbara, CA
David completed the 1987 RAAM (Race Across America), a 3,000-mile event.

"Thanks for the opportunity to give some input, Harry. You asked me if I liked the book. Wrong question. Will it make a difference in the way I manage my life? Well, glad you asked.

"On Tuesday when you called me I was out riding my bike (not interval training, mind you, but I was riding), and the following day I spent an hour and a half in the gym (including some intervals during my thirty minutes on the treadmill). Get the book finished soon so I can buy a copy and keep up the motivation! The chapter on the brain was a blockbuster and the highlight of a very enjoyable book."

— Mark Tonnesen, Retired Mortgage Insurance CEO and Banking Executive, Estero, FL

"I thought I knew a lot about aerobic fitness, the brain and motivation. After all, I've spent a large part of the past twenty-five years running, hiking, biking and working out in the gym, trying to stay young. Your book is helping me get to the next level.

"I have a confession to make. I've been sharing your book, a little at a time, with a young man, twenty years old, who is a drug addict. My hope is that he will take some of your human interest stories to heart as he struggles to get his life back on track."

— George Owens, Retired Senior Vice President, Smith Barney, Boston, MA

"I think that Harry Gaines has written what will be a little jewel of a book. I found it quite readable. The information flows so that the reader wants to keep reading. I kept reading when I should have been doing something else. In fact, at the end of the first chapter I wanted to sign up for his program!

"He writes with enthusiasm — and it's contagious. One of his goals is to motivate people and get them to *move!* He achieves that, no question. This is a book that is a 'good read' as they say, but it is also packed with a wealth of information.

"One of the main goals with the students that I tutor is to make reading interesting and *fun*. I think that he writes with the same purpose, and that's what will be the key to the success of his book."

— Betty Martin, Retired English Teacher, Poway, CA

"After reading your manuscript I changed my priorities of what's important in my life. Daily exercise now comes first. I have to force myself to take a day off every six to eight days. I do strength training more often and continue to ramp up my pace with intervals on the elliptical machine. At the supermarket I pay more attention to product label disclosures (fat, additives, and sugars). I'm anxious to see the book published so I can share it with friends and colleagues."

— John Allison, Owner, John Farley Clothiers, Newburyport, MA

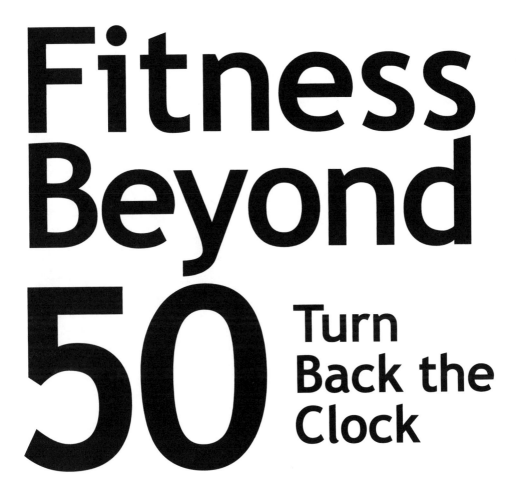

Fitness Beyond

50

Turn Back the Clock

Harry H. Gaines

Achieve Health, Energy and Fitness — At Any Age!

Fitness Beyond 50

Turn Back the Clock

Harry H. Gaines

Langdon Street Press
Minneapolis, MN

Langdon Street Press
212 3rd Avenue North, Suite 290
Minneapolis, MN 55401
612.455.2293
www.langdonstreetpress.com

ISBN-13: 978-1-936782-86-4
LCCN: 2012930119

Distributed by Itasca Books

Cover Design and Typeset by Melanie Shellito

Printed in the United States of America

To Deb, Michael and Michelle — my favorite people.

FOREWORD

"What, and Harry who?" were the first questions I had for my college roommate, Art, when he asked me to assist his friend who was writing a book about fitness for people over fifty. The "what" was because I thought there were enough fitness books out there, why another, and why for those over fifty? And "Who is Harry Gaines?" I had never met nor heard of him. It turned out I was in for a very pleasant experience.

Harry Gaines has turned a personal interest into a passion. He experienced the physical, mental and emotional rewards of engagement in regular physical activity and decided to research what was a good approach to maximize the benefits. The more he looked the more he realized that sound advice and motivational insights for those entering, or in, their retirement stage of life are lacking.

In a thoughtful and thought-provoking manner, Harry explains why it is not too late for those over fifty to obtain the physical and mental benefits derived from physical fitness. He delivers his message clearly and uses numerous real people examples as support. The science and psychology underlying the benefits of engagement in regular physical activity are sound and easy to understand.

As the "Baby Boomers" approach retirement, the "never-too-late" message is germane. What strikes me as particularly good about this book is that it is motivational. The health benefits of physical activity and fitness in reducing cardiovascular, diabetes, obesity and bone density risks are well known and are covered in this book. Harry has also included recent research regarding the benefits of exercise on reducing mental decline associated with aging.

We all are aging, many of us are retiring and there are things we can do to make the latter stages of our circle of life enjoyable and fulfilling. Although we can't stop aging we can affect some of the changes associated with it, and by doing so improve the quality and longevity of our lives. Harry Gaines explains this and does us all a service by presenting it to us in this engaging book.

Roger Kelton, Ph.D.
Former Chair, School of Kinesiology and Health Science
York University
Toronto, Ontario, Canada

PLEASE TELL YOUR FRIENDS

If you like my book I hope you'll share that view with your friends. The success of a book like mine benefits enormously from word-of-mouth marketing. Someone will read it, like it and decide that it's useful information for their friends and relatives who need some education and motivation to get in shape. Some of those readers will read it, take action and share it with others. Ordering it is easy — just go to my website, www.fitnessbeyondfifty.com, or you can order from Amazon, Barnes & Noble or Google Books.

CONTENTS

Youth's Wasted on the Young. A Hypothetical Physical Exam. The Reality.

Where Are We? Who am I? Who's the Audience? Why Did I Write This
Book? The Role of Friends. Relentlessly Nudging. A River Runs Through
It. What's the Reason? What Are the Goals? Leading the Duck. Signing
Up. Signing Up Agreement.

Return on Investment. BMI's Not the Whole Story. There's Fat and
There's Fat. Be a Role Model. For Golfers Only. Limitations. If You Quit,
Don't Give Up. I'm Just Too Busy! But Golf's More Fun. An Alternative
to One Game. Only for Those Who Don't Exercise. Try This. Timing's
Everything. What's the End Game? It Gets to Be Fun. It's Not Just in the
Genes. Check Out Your Life. Let's Review.

I'm Just Not Motivated. Intrinsic or Extrinsic? A Formula for Success.
Let's Get Real. Fear as Motivation. The Curve of Pistophenes. Every Day
in Every Way, I'm Getting Better and Better. Find an Action Trigger.
Paint a Picture — In Your Mind. The Power of the Written Word. Setting
Goals. Goal Summary. Reward Yourself. What's a Habit? I Have a Dream.
Self-Efficacy and Exercise. Retrain Your Brain. Deciding. Do Your Best.
Let's Review.

PROLOGUE: THE PAST, PRESENT AND FUTURE

We all have three phases of our life: the past, the present and the future. We can't change the past; all we can do is learn from it. We can act in the present and determine our future. I'll use an analogy, planning for a vacation, to provide insight into the focus of this book.

A PLANNED OR IMPROMPTU VACATION

We all like to take vacations. Many of us spend lots of time talking about where we want to go and then making the arrangements — airline reservations, hotels, maybe engaging a tour company for a big trip. It's called planning; several studies have shown that planning is more fun for many people than the actual vacation.

Did you see the movie *Bucket List*, starring Jack Nicholson and Morgan Freeman? In the movie they were two guys with incurable diseases who traveled together, completing their list of places they always wanted to see before they "kicked the bucket." Frequently when we mention some place we've visited a friend will say, "That's on my bucket list." They're thinking years ahead about where they want to go.

Suppose we do it a different way. Rather than going through so much planning, why don't we start our vacation by just putting some clothes in a suitcase along with our toiletries and then get in our car with our significant other and drive away? Once we're out of the driveway we can start talking about where we want to go, whether we're going to drive or fly and where we should make hotel reservations.

Your response to this plan would likely be, "Harry, have you lost it? I really look forward to my vacations and I even enjoy planning them. You think I'm going to blow it by doing what you're proposing?" You'd have a good point and I'd agree with you. I wouldn't do it this way either.

Then help me understand why so many of us do exactly that with planning a much more important trip — the rest of our life.

Our life frequently manages us rather than the other way around. Too many haven't spent time thinking about the critical issues of fitness and health. We haven't considered what we'd like to be doing when we're in our seventies and eighties and what we need to do now to ensure that we're healthy enough to do those things. Once we get started, planning our life can be fun also.

Hopefully this book will help you take charge of your life. Put fitness and health at the top of your bucket list.

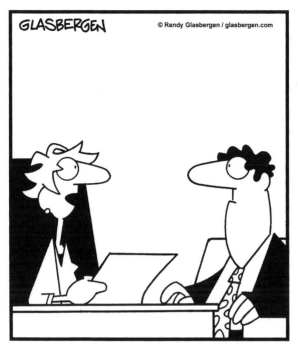

"We have an excellent employee health plan: we built our parking garage 2 miles away from the office!"

INTRODUCTION

"When it comes to reversing the aging process, nothing touches exercise."
—Bob Greene, author and personal trainer for Oprah Winfrey

YOUTH'S WASTED ON THE YOUNG

What George Bernard Shaw actually said was, "Youth is a wonderful thing. What a crime to waste it on children." Physically active youths get away with almost anything in the food department. They seem to be able to eat what they want and in whatever quantities they want.

A physically active youth equals high metabolism. They burn all of that food they put in their mouths. Aside from the physical activity they also have energy going into their growth.

As with all ages, physical activity's an important part of the energy equation.

Inactive youths who eat a lot become overweight or even obese. Those youths have a much harder time reversing it later as their bodies have already adapted to fat formation.

As we mature into adulthood we often change from physically active youths into, in too many cases, physically inactive adults. For a variety of reasons, as people age, their physical activity drops dramatically. They get a job and work hard at a career, get married, have kids and don't have time — or take the time — for exercise. Many keep eating at or close to the input of their former physically active life.

Add two to three pounds a year for thirty years or more and you have too many of today's adults. Thirty-two-inch waists morph into forty-two inches — it happens slowly but steadily. An acquaintance was a top swimmer in college, but forty years later you wouldn't know it to look at him as he's got a few bowling balls around his middle. The same is true for a former nationally ranked tennis player who today is obese. Another friend who played football and baseball at a Big Ten university who's in superb condition laments the poor condition of most of his former teammates of fifty years ago.

What about those of us who were recreational athletes? Too many have fallen victim to the same problem. Singles tennis and pickup basketball games are a thing of the past. Some women give up after having children or perhaps later in midlife.

Many go on a diet periodically to correct the errors of their years, an action that rarely works. Once they lose the weight they go off the diet and gain it back. Only five percent of those who go on a diet keep it off, a sad number.

A friend went for a physical and was told he had problems due to being overweight and physically inactive: high blood pressure and the first stages of type 2 diabetes. He's smart and disciplined in many ways. He got serious, signed up for a diet program and was absolutely religious at adherence. In less than a year, he dropped over fifty pounds and was a shadow of his old self, and looked great. A year later, he'd put it all back on — and then some. I praised him effusively on the way down but have stayed away from any comment about the trip back up. He failed to include exercise as part of his program and also went on a diet — a temporary "fix" — instead of making a lifestyle change.

A HYPOTHETICAL PHYSICAL EXAM

This is not a true story, rather an example of what can happen to many of us. Let's suppose I'm sixty and go in for my annual physical. I've known Dr. Lee, my primary care physician, for many years.

Dr. Lee's completed the exam and has gone to check on test results. He's come back and says, "Harry, I've got all of your tests in now. You're doing OK; not great, but OK. We're controlling your cholesterol with a statin and you're tolerating it just fine; the same for your blood pressure medicine. I think we've got you on the right medications. You're carrying too much weight, as you know. You'd feel better if you lost at least thirty pounds. I know it's not easy, but it sure would help your cholesterol, triglycerides and blood pressure, plus reduce your chances of getting type 2 diabetes.

"I have a lot of senior patients and over the last twenty years I've been seeing some patterns. I've also been attending some seminars on gerontology, since that's become a major part of my practice. I read that 10,000 people are turning sixty-five every day. Recently I thought of a new way of talking to older adults about their health and you're one of the first to hear it. Let's see what you think.

"Suppose that you have two doors to choose from: A or B. Which door you choose will determine your general health and physical activity for the rest of your life.

"Door A is the track you're on now. You play golf several times a week, riding in a cart. You walk the dog a short distance in the morning and evening, maybe ten minutes each time. You like red meat, cheese, French fries and some other foods heavy in saturated fat. You don't gorge yourself but you don't exercise a ton of restraint. You like a pre-dinner cocktail and a glass or two of wine with dinner.

"The good news is that you're likely to be around for another twenty years. The other good news is that you're likely to be OK through your sixties. The bad news is that I can't say that about your seventies and eighties, if you make it that far.

"The patients I see now in their seventies, with life patterns similar to yours, are beginning to have some problems; some lots of them. Many are experiencing coordination problems and are finding it difficult to continue playing golf as much, plus they're frustrated that they can't hit the ball very far. Some are having difficulty with memory and sentence structure — they just don't think as clearly as they used to. They've developed mild cognitive impairment, a precursor to dementia or maybe Alzheimer's.

"I try to interest them in exercise but it's a struggle. They've never been into that and they find it hard to change. Changing their diet is also a challenge. Their future isn't real bright. There's a slow downhill progression that, given their lifestyle, is unavoidable. We don't have any pills for that.

"Let's go to Door B. Going through this door requires a lifestyle change, both in exercise and diet. It's not a trivial commitment. It means three or four days a week of aerobics, a minimum of thirty minutes, preferably an hour, and two days a week of serious strength training. This produces stronger muscles, bones, ligaments and tendons plus improved coordination, which helps avoid injury or falls. It means devoting at least five hours a week to exercise.

"Compared to what you do now this may seem to be a lot of exercise. It's five hours of 112 awake hours per week, assuming eight hours per night of sleep, less than five percent of your week. It's a commitment to better health and a better quality of life that requires five percent of your time. What a bargain.

"It means that you stop eating junk food and significantly reduce the amount of red meat. I can outline in more detail a healthy eating lifestyle. It also means reducing the cocktails and wine to a smaller number.

"That's the bad news or good news, depending upon how you look at it. But the good news for sure is that you dramatically increase your chances of leading an active life through your eighties, and I mean by a lot. And the other good news is that I think you'll find the exercise and healthier eating enjoyable, once you get into it.

"I compare it to quitting smoking, which virtually all of my patients have done. They know that smoking shortens their life, both in quality and quantity. The opposite can be said for starting an exercise program. Both are hard and both are very rewarding.

"And here's the other really good news; research over the last decade shows that exercise has an enormous impact on brain function. Those who exercise regularly have a much lower incidence of those problems we don't like to talk or even think about. This, to me, is the real elephant in the room."

THE REALITY

I'm not really sixty; I'm seventy-three, as I'm writing this. I didn't experience the physical exam described above. I'm fortunate to be in good shape, but it didn't have to be that way and it didn't happen without effort and commitment.

I'm writing this book for my friends as well as those I've never met but would like to through these pages. Maybe the following chapters pertain to you as well as friends of yours whose companionship you'd like to enjoy for many years to come.

I hope you enjoy reading this book as much as I did writing it.

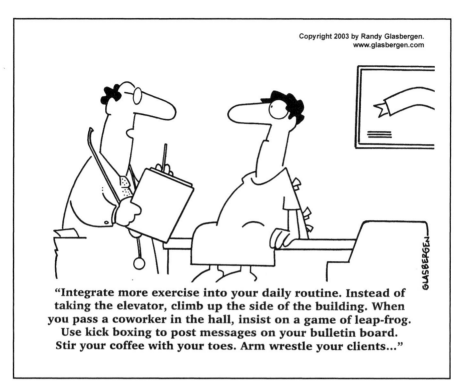

"Integrate more exercise into your daily routine. Instead of taking the elevator, climb up the side of the building. When you pass a coworker in the hall, insist on a game of leap-frog. Use kick boxing to post messages on your bulletin board. Stir your coffee with your toes. Arm wrestle your clients..."

CHAPTER ONE — LET'S GET STARTED

"This journey of a thousand miles begins with a single step."
—*Lao Tzu, 604 BC–531 BC.*

WHERE ARE WE?

The poor physical condition of much of the adult population in the United States is disturbing. The nation's health is the worst it's ever been.

Very few adults do any moderate or strenuous exercise on a regular basis. The lack of exercise isn't restricted to any particular group. You know as well as I do — no matter where you go in this country, at all levels of our society, we see people in all age groups who are significantly overweight or obese. Health authorities and the media constantly bemoan the fact that this country is getting fatter.

Among adults (age twenty or over), sixty-eight percent are overweight; thirty-four percent of those overweight are in the obese category — that's a body mass index (BMI) of thirty or more. BMI is a method of measurement used by health professionals to evaluate health based on height and weight.

Obesity rates in the United States have increased sixty percent in the past ten years. More than fifty percent of adults don't engage in enough physical activity to make a difference in their health.

The August 2011 issue of *Scientific American* mentioned that sixty-two percent of adults in North, Central and South America are overweight, the highest rate of any global region. The lowest is Southeast Asia at fourteen percent.

How and why did we achieve this appalling state? It makes sense that most adults would see the wisdom of taking care of themselves so that they can lead a longer, healthier life and do the things they enjoy. How could they possibly want to spend their last years, which should be an enjoyable and productive period of their life, shuffling around with a walker or, worse yet, in a wheelchair at an assisted living facility?

We're certainly smart enough and are continuously bombarded with information (magazines, newspapers, TV, the internet) telling us what we should do. But many of us can't seem to find the motivation to make a change in our lives.

Many adults I know were competitive athletes in high school and college: swimming, playing tennis, football, baseball, basketball or running track. Some are relatively trim but not even close to being fit aerobically, nor is their muscular conditioning any better. Too many are overweight and look like they never do anything more strenuous than riding in a golf cart. What happened?

Exercise never made it onto their list of priorities. They had few role models as most of their parents rarely did anything strenuous. To be fair to our parents, many were too busy trying to survive during the Great Depression, fighting WWII, then starting a career and raising a family. It was a different time and they had little time to focus on health — it was more about survival. The information about fitness available in the fifties, sixties and seventies was a fraction of what's out there today.

One factor that's changed is the type of work we do or did compared to our forefathers. Most of them probably worked standing up or doing physical labor — working in a factory or on a farm. Our careers involved more time sitting behind a desk. We've become a sedentary society.

Is it too late? Once a man or woman reaches their fifties, then into their sixties and seventies, have they missed the golden ring? Consciously or subconsciously, many may think so. "Why bother? I'm too old and too out of shape to make a difference. Why not relax, enjoy life as long as I can. When it's over, it's over; that's my fate."

Lots of research and actual case histories show that it's never too late. Every time I hear those last few words I think of Churchill's famous 1940 speech ending with "We shall never surrender!" When it comes to taking care of ourselves, we shouldn't either.

And here's the really good news: the worse shape you're in now, the more quickly you'll see improvement. Imagine the worst being the fastest to improve. They have the most to gain and it shows up fairly quickly.

Our fate is not set in stone. There's no reason that we can't become more aerobically fit and strong — two different goals — if we'll make a commitment to do it. Provided that Mother Nature doesn't trip us up with a seriously debilitating illness, we don't ever have to surrender.

Coaches in sports and the arts teach the practice of visualization. Golf instructors have you visualize the shot you're going to hit, the ball flight, where it's going to land. Then they have you hit it.

Visualize what you can become if you commit to becoming more active and to improving your physical fitness. Use this to get over the hurdles of lethargy, lack of habit or motivation. Think about the "new you."

WHO AM I?

I'm a guy in his seventies who's been exercising most of his life. I enjoy being in good physical condition. I gain a lot of satisfaction from time in the gym and on my bike. There are days when I'd prefer to take it easy versus going for a bike ride or doing strength training, but over the years I've figured out how to overcome those feelings — just go and do it. I always feel better after and this helps the next time I waver. I also have several action triggers I use, a concept I'll explain soon.

Who I'm not is an M.D., Ph.D., kinesiologist, exercise physiologist or personal trainer. Multiple individuals in each of those categories have read this book in draft form and certified the accuracy of the science, among other things. Rather, I'm a retired publishing executive who likes doing research on exercise topics and who discovered late in life that he's a decent writer. At least that's what my reviewers have told me, and I hope you agree.

When cycling I frequently ride with a group. The peer pressure to show up is strong. Having others to do exercise with is so important that there's a separate chapter on that topic. The golf pro Gary Player is famous for saying, "The harder

I work, the luckier I get." For us it can be, "The harder I exercise, the stronger and more fit I get, plus the better I feel."

When I meet someone new they often say something like, "You're retired?" I tell them that I have a part-time job; they usually ask what it is. I explain, "Taking care of myself. I spend ten hours a week doing the things that will keep me healthy and fit — cycling, strength training and general exercises. As long as I show up for my part-time job I'll be able to do the things I like to do for the rest of my life."

Do you have to do ten hours a week to get results? No. I enjoy cycling and a ride today is at least two hours, often three or more — that's my choice. A session at the gym is about one hour twice a week, so ten or more turns out to be a good number for me. You can obtain excellent results with fewer hours. We'll discuss how many later.

Develop a program, stick with it, see the benefits and convince relatives and friends to do the same. Like missionaries, one soul at a time gets converted.

WHO'S THE AUDIENCE?

One audience is men and women over fifty who do some exercise currently but not as much as they likely know they should. Many are seeking education and motivation. A short and simple presentation with lots of success stories is appealing. Stories of super athletes and their prowess can be intimidating, but many of them do want to raise the bar.

Men and women who currently do significant exercise regularly are also good candidates for education and motivation. Many are likely open to more complexity — doing more and working out harder. They may not fully understand the value of really pushing themselves.

Men and women who do not now exercise, never have and have little motivation to do so are still candidates. Some may become strong candidates as a result of a catastrophic event — a heart attack, a frank discussion with a doctor they trust or the death or incapacity of a close friend due to poor health and lack of exercise. Motivation may come from seeing others who are physically active or a desire to do more activities with their children or grandchildren.

The only person who can motivate anyone to do something hard, like exercise, is themselves. Success stories of people in all categories are included.

WHY DID I WRITE THIS BOOK?

This book got started as a result of my serendipitously meeting Scott, a guy from a fitness company. We talked, shared a few emails and he asked me to write some articles for his company's fitness blog. I wrote several and also sent them to some friends, who encouraged me to write a book. I also wrote some articles for our local fitness center newsletter in SW Florida and got similar comments about writing a book.

I thought about it and decided the challenge of learning enough to be able to write a book was really appealing. Much of the writing has been an enormous amount of fun. I'll meet someone, tell them what I'm doing and they'll tell a story. I'll go home, write it, send it to them for review and add their comments. Many of the stories are based on personal experiences with friends over the years. Many are written by friends who've read parts of the manuscript and added a story of their own.

The main reasons for writing it were:

- I have a passion for exercise, fitness, healthy eating and staying connected. I'd like to motivate others to take action in order to live a healthier and more active life.

- I decided that, in my early seventies, I wanted to do something hard, and writing a book qualifies. Norman Maclean was a model; his story is coming up shortly. Maclean was ahead of me as he'd written a terrific book before doing one that was hard.

I hope you enjoy this book. Even if you like it, only you can decide to make the lifestyle changes required to implement the ideas in the book. No amount of cajoling, threatening or pleading by any third party will do it.

People get serious about fitness and health for a variety of reasons. One friend got going to avoid dying. Another took action out of embarrassment at being out-cycled by a friend twenty years his senior. A third wanted to improve his memory before it was too late. Al Roker made a commitment to his father on his father's deathbed. Al's had some relapses, but as of this writing he's down from 340 to 200 pounds and is exercising regularly.

So whatever your motivation — fear, peer pressure, promises, a desire to get healthy again — I hope you do it. The rewards are enormous. I first heard the phrase, "Today is the first day of the rest of your life" over forty years ago. It's still true today.

Bill Y read this section and told me a line he remembered: "Retirement — the next stage in life devoted to taking good care of you."

WHY-TO

I was discussing the book with my son Michael and he asked, "Dad, what's different about your book?" I said, "My book is not a 'how-to' book about specific exercises; it's focused on education and motivation. The goal is to get readers to understand what they're missing by not exercising and eating healthy and what they'll gain if they do." He said, "Then it's a 'why-to' book."

THE ROLE OF FRIENDS

During the process of writing this book I've benefited from the constructive comments of a number of friends as well as friends of friends. This includes several specialists in exercise physiology, one of whom was chair of a large department of kinesiology and health science at a major university in Canada, a number of M.D.s, Ph.D.s in various areas of science, plus friends very experienced in exercise who could offer a reader's perspective. The scientists and M.D.s have confirmed that the science in the book is correct and the others have hopefully kept me on the right path in explaining the science to the typical reader.

Frequently the reviewers responded with interesting comments or stories about their own experiences. That's why you'll see a lot of stories beginning with the first name of the individual who wrote it. I've always liked stories as a way to reinforce and remember concepts and ideas. They also can provide motivation.

RELENTLESSLY NUDGING

Nudge: Improving Decisions About Health, Wealth, and Happiness by Thaler and Sunstein was published in 2008. It's a book about behavioral economics. They demonstrate how thoughtful "choice architecture" can be established to nudge us in beneficial directions.

One example is about women deciding whether to join a 401K program at a new job. If they're given a choice of whether or not to join, about thirty percent sign up. However, if they are automatically enrolled unless they elect to opt out, about eighty percent do it.

I hired Art as a sales representative in Southern California in 1968. We've been friends ever since and now live near each other half of the year in SW Florida. During the process of writing this book Art came to my house one day and we reviewed chapters of the manuscript. After a day's work we were having a glass of wine prior to going out for dinner. We were talking about the approach of the book and Art said:

"Harry, when you were a sales manager over forty years ago you used to relentlessly nudge those of us who worked with you to do better. I think you're doing the same thing in this book; relentlessly nudging the reader to do more."

As soon as he said it I thought of Thaler and Sunstein's book, which I read several years ago. Their goal was to inform people of how thoughtful choices can benefit them.

Over the course of writing this book I've listened to adults, both men and women, who've said something like, "I know I should do more exercise; I know it's good for me. I just need something to get me going. Maybe reading your manuscript will help." The good news is that a high percentage of those who've read it in draft form have taken action.

I hope I'll be able to "relentlessly nudge" you into taking action. The goal is to get you to make thoughtful choices that will benefit you for the rest of your life.

A NUDGE STORY

Rick M agreed to review the first seven chapters of this book and asked if he could send a copy to his mother Betty, a retired schoolteacher in her early eighties. I told him I'd love to have her comments. Betty wrote a very positive review and then sent me the following email:

"A few minutes after I wrote Rick with my comments I had an afterthought. Here's what I wrote: "Hi again, Rick. Last week we were in Costco and I was standing and looking longingly at the chocolate-covered almonds. We've had them before and they're outstandingly good. I was about to reach for a jar of them when Harry Gaines whispered in my ear and I walked away. Can you believe that?"

Congratulations, Betty, on a fine display of willpower. If my book happens to reduce the sale of chocolate-covered almonds at Costco, so be it.

A RIVER RUNS THROUGH IT

Norman Maclean wrote a marvelous book, *A River Runs Through It*, the first work of fiction ever published by the University of Chicago Press. It's a great story, beautifully written; Robert Redford produced and directed an equally good movie. Maclean was a professor of English at the University of Chicago, where he held the William Rainey Harper Chair.

In 1993, he published a less well-known book, *Young Men and Fire*, the story of fifteen firefighters for the U. S. Forest Service who parachuted in to fight a fire in Montana and were killed. Maclean had to learn a great deal about the science and mathematics of fires, not an area of expertise for him. I remember reading the passage where he said he wanted to do something hard. He described in some detail what he had to do to write the book and he then said, "And it was."

For those who've never done it, starting a serious exercise program falls into the category of something really hard. It has the potential of being enormously rewarding, but it's hard to commit and get started. And, once started, it's hard to keep showing up. Many give up before the habit is formed.

JOHN F. KENNEDY

The following is from a speech by President John F. Kennedy on September 12, 1962, at Rice University Stadium:

"We choose to go to the moon. We choose to go to the moon in this decade and do the other things, not because they are easy, but because they are hard, because that goal will serve to organize and measure the best of our energies and skills, because that challenge is one that we are willing to accept, one we are unwilling to postpone, and one which we intend to win, and the others, too."

I think that qualifies as something hard. It makes our need to take care of ourselves seem pretty easy, doesn't it?

WHAT'S THE REASON?

Getting into the heads of a representative group of men and women as to why they're not fit isn't easy, but some of the likely issues are:

- **Lack of Knowledge** — Many people are unaware of the benefits of a vigorous exercise program. Equally important, they're unaware of the consequences of not exercising. They don't realize that many diseases — high blood pressure, type 2 diabetes, heart disease, even some cancers, can be prevented — not delayed — by exercise. They may look at their partner across the breakfast table from them, in the same boat, and think, "Why bother?" Even if you already have some of the health conditions listed above, you can improve or even eliminate them with a serious exercise program.

- **Motivation** — Starting an exercise program when you've never done it, particularly when you're in your fifties, sixties or seventies, is hard. You feel strange, out of place, uncertain of what to do and how to do it. This topic is so important that I devote a chapter to it.

- **Priorities** — Adults have many priorities. Some are still working while others spend time reading, doing volunteer work, being with grandkids, playing golf, maybe working a part-time job. As one said not long ago, "I'm so busy!" Developing and sticking with a serious exercise program just never made the list.

- **Habit** — We devote our lives to our job and family and "don't have time for exercise." I suggest that we don't take time. We never got into the habit of regular exercise.

- **Rationalization** — Many look around and see that their friends are not any more fit than they are. If it's such a big deal, why aren't their friends doing it? They've got lots of company. Some think that walking — actually strolling — around the neighborhood for a half-hour with their dog or going to the gym twice a week but never working hard enough to produce real results is enough.

- **Timing** — Consciously or subconsciously, we may think that it's too late. The cards are already dealt and no new hand is available.

WHAT ARE THE GOALS?

The goals of this book will be to deal with these issues and try to motivate more adults to take more action:

- Get started

- If possible, hire a trainer (more on this later)

- Develop a program

- Set short-term goals and work to achieve them

- Then set higher goals

- Keep records

- Read material on fitness and eating well

- Join — or even initiate — a support group

- Talk to others who exercise and listen to what they do

- Stick with it until it becomes a habit

We'll deal with these and other issues in more detail later in the book.

STILL WORKING

John said: "I'm not sure what percent of the book speaks to folks who are retired but you want to make sure you also focus on guys like me, now sixty-seven, who still work. We need to do all this and still fit it in our schedule.

"I recently joined Planet Fitness and started using the elliptical trainer — it feels great, better than walking fast on the treadmill. The best thing about the elliptical is that I can increase my speed by twenty percent over the treadmill. Every five minutes I do a one-minute interval going as fast as I can. I weigh 158 pounds, about what I weighed when I got out of the Air Force in 1969, and my waist is thirty-two inches. I'm getting ready for ski season."

GOT THE RELIGION

Pat, fifty years old, has a busy life as a wife, mother of three children and managing director for a private investment firm. Still, she manages to maintain a regular, rigorous exercise program. She recently sent this email:

"I got the exercise 'religion' about three years ago after recognizing that the investment made in working out would have huge benefits as I get older. It's pretty simple: you just have to move your body and circulate the blood to all your muscles, especially your brain. Just as you wouldn't keep a Maserati in the garage or it would rust and not function properly, you need to exercise regularly so your body works well.

"Many people think exercise won't make a difference. The problem with this complacency is the inability to see the benefits or at least avoid the very unpleasant outcomes related to stagnation. There is such a better path as we all age. Whether you focus on the 'carrot' — for me skiing into old age, or the 'stick' — avoiding illness, medicines and worse, you just need to make a commitment to doing some form of exercise regularly.

"There are many days when I don't feel like going to run, bike or the gym, but I make myself go because I know I'll feel good afterward. I feel a sense of accomplishment after a workout and the positive energy lasts the whole day. I've now gotten to the point where I get frustrated when I don't work out.

"Exercise doesn't just make me stronger and healthier; it substantially improves my mood and attitude. I'm so much happier when I work out. I'm more calm, less emotional, much more at peace and able to get important things done. Exercise helps me focus, gives me confidence and makes me strong physically and mentally. My interactions with my husband and kids are so much better and I know I've inspired them too. My husband and I are biking together and my teenagers run and work out. I've noticed positive changes in all of us."

I was listening to NPR recently. A survey of one thousand adults yielded the result that eighty-five percent of those surveyed thought they were leading a healthier life, exercising more and eating better, than a year ago. But they thought only twenty percent of their friends and relatives were doing the same.

The survey said that the biggest obstacles to doing more were time, resources and motivation. Those of us who are retired have only one real obstacle: motivation. Lack of motivation can be overcome, but it's up to us to change it. Those not retired can overcome the time and resources obstacles, provided they develop motivation.

A LIFETIME OF EXERCISE

Ted lives in a nearby community in SW Florida. He knew that I was looking for stories about women who exercise regularly, so when he saw Joan at a social gathering he spotted her as a likely candidate. Joan obviously takes care of herself. When I called Joan, then seventy-eight, I asked her how long she's been exercising. Her response was, "All of my life!"

Over the years Joan has participated in tennis, platform tennis, skiing, golf and exercise classes. Today she walks three miles five times a week, does fitness and strength training one day a week, plus two days of Zumba classes. She's doing some form of exercise virtually every day.

She told me, "I not only enjoy the exercise but also the aftereffects; I feel so good after I do physical activity. I don't understand why others don't get it, why they fail to understand what a positive effect exercise will have on their lives."

Tara Parker-Pope wrote the following in *The New York Times*: "Healthy living doesn't happen at the doctor's office. The road to better health is paved with the small decisions we make every day. It's about the choices we make when we buy groceries, drive our cars and hang out with our kids."

THE MAGIC PILL

My wife Deb and I went on a tour of Egypt and Jordan in the fall of 2010, and had a wonderful time. One of the couples we met was Grant and Maria from Auckland, New Zealand. They were on a five-week vacation in Europe and the Mideast. It always amazes me how Aussies and Kiwis hop around the world like it was their backyard. Of course, anywhere they want to go is a long ways away.

Grant is a doctor in Auckland, what we call a primary care physician. I was fascinated to learn that he has over 2,500 patients and that he doesn't require his patients to make an appointment. They sit in the waiting room until he can see them and he leaves when he's the only person left, often after 9 PM.

Grant is a triathlete. He's also an avid hiker and cyclist who truly believes in the value of exercise. He said that his patients are surprised at how many times he says, no matter what their problem, "Go get some exercise." He views exercise as the "magic pill."

JOHN STEINBECK

Steinbeck is one of my favorite authors. One of his quotes I like is what he said about his good friend Ed Ricketts, who was killed when a train hit his car. Ricketts was his partner on the biology expedition that produced the book, *Log from the Sea of Cortez*, and was the basis for the biologist in *Cannery Row*:

"We had a relationship that just growed and growed."

I thought of it in relation to exercise; the more exercise we do the more our relationship with it grows and grows. It's like spending time with a good friend — we feel better when we do.

LEADING THE DUCK

Over twenty years ago we acquired a small training company that had developed one of the best corporate training programs ever produced. Tod, the founder, is a brilliant original thinker. One day I mentioned a *Business Week* article on marketing to Tod and quoted a sentence from it: "If you're shooting a duck, you don't aim where he is; you aim where he's going to be." Tod's immediate response was, "No, you aim where he should be."

This book is not aimed at where many of you are or where you're going to be, it's aimed at where you should be. There can be a significant difference. Write down on a piece of paper or store in a computer file some vital statistics; your current weight, waist measurement and blood pressure. If you have the data add your blood lipid profile — total cholesterol, HDL, LDL and triglycerides as well as glucose. Add the current date.

If you read this book and decide to implement many of the ideas suggested, you'll make a significant change in your life. A year from now, even sooner, you can be where you should be. You'll look, act and feel like a different person, guaranteed. The vital statistics you wrote down earlier will be very different from your new numbers.

If you're new to a regular exercise program, reading this book can be the first step. Changing your life will require a commitment, determination, persistence and a strong desire to live a long, active, healthy life. Those are all qualities we'd like to instill in our children as well as ourselves. We can be the role model for them as well as for our grandchildren.

I fervently hope you make that decision.

SIGNING UP

Tracy Kidder has written many books. His first, *The Soul of a New Machine*, for which he won a Pulitzer Prize, is a story about building a new computer at a now defunct company, Data General.

Building a new computer required a group of committed professionals, people who agreed to do whatever it took to get the job done no matter the hours. Kidder called it "Signing Up." Once you signed up, everything else took second place. Weekends off were a thing of the past.

Kidder said, "Promising to achieve a nearly impossible schedule was a way of signing up. Signing up required, of course, that you fervently desire the right to build your machine and that you do whatever was necessary for success."

This was a commitment. We talk a lot about commitment — to a job, spouse, family, friends or specific causes. A commitment to taking care of ourself is also important.

One of the big problems adults face in starting an exercise program is signing up. They go to the gym a few times, get discouraged by limited progress, soreness, maybe miss a few days and then it's all over. They never made a true commitment so they don't go back. It never became a habit and they never saw enough results. Getting going again is hard.

When you get started, Sign Up. Go, no matter how you feel. If you have company, tell them you'll be back in an hour or so. Stick with the program.

SIGNING UP AGREEMENT

I want and need to change my life. I want to lead a healthy, active life as long as possible and am committing to doing the things that will make that happen. I recognize that it's totally within my abilities to do so. I'll develop an exercise program and will stick with it. I'll show up, no matter what.

I'll be patient, recognizing that it will take time to see and feel the results. It took me many years to get to where I am now, and I can't expect the changes to be overnight. But, I am confident that they will happen and, once they start, success will breed further success.

I'll keep records, which will further motivate me. I'll write down exercises as I do them and also the aerobic work — cycling, walking, running. Recording the results will help me see and measure progress, which will lead to further progress.

I recognize that every day won't be fun. I also recognize that, even when it's not fun, I will finish feeling better for having done it.

_____ Date:_____

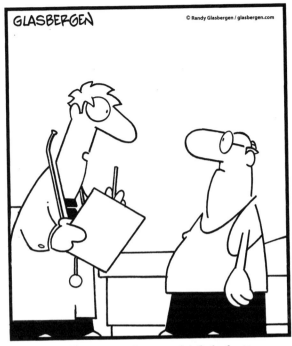

"What fits your busy schedule better,
exercising one hour a day or being
dead 24 hours a day?"

CHAPTER TWO — LIFE'S FULL OF CHOICES

*Craig Venter was the first person to sequence the human genome. Born in 1946,
he said the following in the June 2011 issue of* Men's Journal, *when asked the question,
"How should a man handle getting old?"*

"By fighting it at every stage — mentally, physically. If you start to think of
yourself as old, you will be."

HERE'S WHAT'S COMING

- What can you do to live a longer and healthier life? Is it worth the time required?
- What's BMI?
- What are the different kinds of fat?

- Is it too late for you to make a difference in your life?
- How can you be a role model for your children and their children?
- What if you quit — how do you get started again?
- What if you've never exercised?
- How big a role do genes play?

DALAI LAMA

The Dalai Lama, when asked what surprised him most about humanity, answered, "Man. Because he sacrifices his health in order to make money. Then he sacrifices money to recuperate his health. And then he is so anxious about the future that he does not enjoy the present. The result being that he does not live in the present or the future; he lives as if he is never going to die, and then dies having never really lived."

RETURN ON INVESTMENT

Those who are retired, or close to it, have spent time reviewing their investments. Some have met with a financial planner and asked questions about whether they'll have enough income to cover their needs and wants in retirement. Others choose to do it on their own. They make assumptions about their anticipated return on investment and plan for unanticipated events.

Let's apply that thinking to our fitness and health. What investment are we willing to make in order to significantly increase our chances of living a longer and healthier life?

There are 168 hours in a week. Most of us sleep about eight hours a night, which leaves 112 hours per week available for other activities.

Those who are retired used to spend forty or more hours working. We now have that time available for whatever we choose to do with it. Spending five to ten hours per week exercising equals four and a half percent to nine percent of the available time.

Individuals who exercise regularly are likely to live both a healthier and longer life. *Research has shown that a highly active sixty-five year old adds,*

*on average, 5.7 years of healthy life expectancy — compared to the average
for his or her age.*

Say you're willing to commit to seven hours a week for aerobic and
strength training. It's dramatically less than the time you used to spend
working — less than one day of work.

Gaining an extra 5.7 years of healthy life adds up to 296 weeks or
49,800 hours. Deducting eight hours of sleeping time per day, you've got
33,200 hours of extra time.

Stick with your commitment of seven hours a week for ten years and
you'll have invested 3,640 hours. And for that you have the potential to
gain 33,200 active hours. You're getting back nine times what you invested.

We know that something unforeseen can happen to derail this plan,
not unlike what can happen to our investments. But if someone said to me,
"Harry, I'm asking you to invest $3,640 over ten years; not all at once but
daily over that span. In return I'm going to give you the high probability
of a return of $33,200. Are you interested?" Of course I am. My financial
advisor calculated the annual rate of return — forty-two percent.

What these numbers don't show is how much better your life will be.
You'll feel, look and behave like a different person. You'll be able to do
more things and have a much fuller life.

Most of us choose our financial investments carefully. We weigh the
pros and cons, seek advice and make rational decisions based on the
available information. Why not apply the same quality of thinking to our
fitness and health? What does any amount of wealth do for us personally,
once we're six feet under?

BMI'S NOT THE WHOLE STORY

Body Mass Index (BMI) is a method of body measurement based on height
and weight. BMI is used by health professionals to help determine whether
someone is overweight or not, but it doesn't tell the whole story.

An individual could weigh the same as thirty years ago but have three or four
more inches around the middle; that's fat. They've lost muscle mass and gained fat,
not the right way to go. Muscle weighs more than fat but fat takes up more space.

Another individual who's been doing both aerobic and strength training for years could be above the BMI and still be very healthy — he or she is carrying more heavy muscle but less fat.

Focus on your body fat and be honest about it. There are very fit "overweight" individuals, such as some professional athletes, and there are very unfit "underweight" individuals, such as professional models. Think about your body fat. Three accepted ways to determine your level of fat are:

- Your waist in inches should be no more than half of your height in inches. As you age it's definitely easier to get slimmer than taller.

- Measure around the widest part of the abdomen and around the hips; calculate the waist-to-hip ratio. For men it should be no higher than .90, for women .83.

- Your doctor or a trainer at a gym can perform a skin-fold score based on measurements taken with a caliper at several areas.

> Roger said: "The best method for me is to just look in the mirror. Am I lean? Do I have muscle definition, particularly in my midsection? How does my clothing fit? Do I have extra holes in my belt? Can I see my feet when standing erect? How is my body profile? Am I flabby?"

THERE'S FAT AND THERE'S FAT

There are two type of fat — subcutaneous and visceral.

Subcutaneous fat is located just under the skin. One indication of it is cellulite. It serves as a source of energy during exercise and other periods of intensity and helps cushion our skin against trauma. We all have a good supply of subcutaneous fat.

Visceral fat is located around vital organs in the abdomen. It can take residence in your liver and other organs, get into your muscles and even put a strangle hold on your heart. *It's the one linked to heart disease, high cholesterol, diabetes and strokes.* Having a high percentage of visceral fat is definitely not a good idea.

Individuals with large bellies have too much visceral fat, but even thin people may have an excess of it. The only way to tell for sure is by an MRI test. The best way to limit visceral fat is via exercise. Researchers have shown that those who do little or no exercise have a higher proportion of visceral fat than those who exercise regularly. Those who do some exercise — a minimum of thirty minutes of brisk walking six times a week — can limit the accumulation of additional visceral fat. Those with a more vigorous program can reverse the amount.

SOCIETY'S VIEW OF WEIGHT AND OBESITY

Paul said: "I'm sixty-nine years old and five feet nine inches tall; my highest weight was 236 pounds. I've lost and gained fifty to seventy pounds two or three times in the past fifteen years. I had a heart attack at age sixty-three when I weighed about 210 pounds.

"It's my opinion that society has set itself up incorrectly in its judgment of one's weight. I can't count the number of people who told me that I looked healthy when I weighed 210–220 pounds. When I lose sixty-five to seventy pounds I can't count the number of people who tell me that I am way too skinny, that I don't look healthy.

"When I weigh 165 to 170 pounds my doctor is happy and my cardiologist is happy; yet I'm asked if I'm sick or on chemo. When I weigh 168 I take far less medicine (if any) than when I weigh 220, yet society seems to be severely affected by what it has become used to seeing: an overweight society. They judge the weight of others according to an incorrect notion of what's a healthy weight."

JUST SIT

Bob hired me fresh out of college as a sales rep in the college textbook industry. Fifteen years my senior, he was my mentor and friend for almost fifty years.

He was Juniors Champion in tennis for North and South Carolina, WWII vet in the Pacific, honor graduate of Harvard and played on the tennis team there. A successful corporate executive in publishing, he devoted his life to work. He played recreational tennis after college but not regularly. He got very little exercise and married late in life.

We talked frequently and met for meals for decades after I left the company. I'd talk to him about exercise and get nowhere. His standard response, in that Southern drawl he never lost, was, "Harry, at my age the best thing a man can do is just sit."

He retired in his mid-sixties as a wealthy man. Unfortunately, he spent the last ten years of his life in a nursing home, the last five bedridden due to various problems. He died at age eighty-five. During his active years Bob was always trim and looked fit even though he wasn't. I don't think he had any underlying health problems that led to his deterioration. It's likely that the biggest factor was his lack of exercise.

STAY ACTIVE

Contrast him to Bill E, now eighty-six. Also a WWII vet, he landed at Le Havre, France, in September 1944. After the war he graduated from Cornell, played on the tennis team there and has been an athlete all of his life.

Bill plays golf three times a week, rides his bike five to ten miles several times and does core exercises at home. He looks seventy and acts sixty. His wife, twenty years younger, struggles to keep up with him. Bill writes musical lyrics and is working to get some songs published. He found a singer, composer and studio and has recorded a number of his songs. He's well-read, interesting and interested in others.

My son Michael, forty-two, spent an hour with him and was fascinated. He couldn't stop telling me what a great guy Bill is. Sometimes when I'm playing golf with Bill I'll look over and think, "My partner landed in France in 1944, when I was seven years old."

Recently Bill learned that he had a swollen aorta and needed to have open heart surgery. Bill's cardiologist was comfortable recommending he have the surgery, even at his age, because he's in excellent condition as a result of his lifelong exercise. The good news is that he's had the surgery and is on the road to recovery.

His wife Margarita said: "I have to add that the doctors said Bill would never have done so well had he not been fit. Most of the heart patients we saw were obese."

Bob chose Door A many years ago; Bill chose Door B, also many years ago. How come there are so many more Bobs than Bills? And can we do anything about it? Is it possible to get adults to get with a program that will allow them to enjoy a longer, healthier life? Or do they just not care?

START ANYTIME

Pat sent me this story about her mother, Ilona: "Maybe one good example is to talk about the fact that you can start anytime. I got my mom to exercise when she was seventy-six.

"She read *Younger Next Year* (a book Pat recommended) and when we were on vacation in the summer in Avalon, NJ, we started going for walks. We walked each day and I got her to go longer each time.

"When she returned home she kept it up and walked three miles daily. This is a woman who never exercised in any formal way. As a youth she had to walk miles and miles after school, getting to her home from the train in Hungary.

"Her blood pressure had been high prior to walking but she stubbornly refused medicine. After she started walking for awhile, her blood pressure decreased substantially and she didn't have the need for medicine anymore. It made a big impact.

"She had a fall a year ago but I think it would have been a longer and harder recovery had she not been in shape. She still walks and does strength training exercises at home at seventy-nine."

THE FOUNTAIN OF YOUTH

The *Bucks County Magazine* published a special section in their summer 2011 issue, Annual Guide to Healthy Living. One of the more interesting articles was "The Fountain of Youth" by Margo Aramian Ragan. One of her quotes was from Dr. Mary Ann Forciea, medical director at a local independent and assisted living community: "When a resident comes to me to talk about physical fitness, I am thrilled. I always encourage the individual. No matter how frail a person may be, exercise will be a benefit."

One of the stories was about Dan, a patient of hers. He was fifty pounds overweight, had tried lots of diets but had given up on losing the weight. While he'd never smoked or abused alcohol, he also had never done any exercise. When he was told that he needed to begin an exercise program he said that, at seventy-four, it would be too dangerous for him to do that. He added, "Dr. Forciea told me that the more dangerous thing for me to do was to continue sitting at my computer."

Dan started doing aerobics, strength training, balance and stretching exercises. He now works out six days a week and has, over two years, almost reached his goal of losing fifty pounds. He said, "The fitness program has changed my life. It's the best investment I've ever made."

BE A ROLE MODEL

Recently I had a meeting with Regan, a charming young woman who's Vice President of Field Operations for the American Heart Association in SW Florida. She shocked me when she said that the predictions are that the current kids in elementary and high school are projected to be the first generation that will have a shorter life expectancy than their parents. Here's a quote from their website:

"Today, about one in three American kids and teens is overweight or obese, nearly triple the rate in 1963. Among children today, obesity is causing a broad range of health problems that previously weren't seen until adulthood. These include high blood pressure, type 2 diabetes and elevated blood cholesterol levels. There are also psychological effects: obese children are more prone to low self-esteem, negative body image and depression. And excess weight at young ages has been linked to higher and earlier death rates in adulthood."

In terms of fitness and healthy eating, what type of role model are you for your children and grandchildren? What type of role model would you like to be?

FOR GOLFERS ONLY

Some of us have friends who play lots of golf and do little else. Most, out of requirement or choice, ride in a cart. The level of exercise involved is low.

Let's say someone plays five times a week, which many do. That's about twenty-five hours of time, counting a warming-up period.

A number of golfer friends have mentioned that they likely won't be playing much once they reach their mid-seventies because of anticipated physical problems due to their health. That, of course, is due to their lack of real exercise. Suppose that a golfer made a choice; instead of playing five times a week he or she played three and devoted seven hours of the extra ten now available to real exercise — aerobics, anaerobics, core exercises and strength training.

Remember at the beginning of this chapter — a highly active person in their mid-sixties lives an average of 5.7 years longer. If from age sixty-seven to eighty they devoted seven hours a week for exercise, that's about 4,700 hours. If they pick up an extra 5.7 years of golf time, playing three days a week, five hours total per round, that's 4,450 hours of golf.

Wait, you say; he or she has invested 4,700 hours to get 4,450 hours. That's not such a good deal. But, remember — an extra 5.7 years of enjoying their favorite sport is a huge deal. Plus the total extra time of an active, healthy life, deducting eight hours per day for sleep, is 33,200 hours. That seems like a mighty fine investment to me.

LIMITATIONS

What if you have some health issues that you feel may limit your ability to do the things discussed in this book? While you certainly want to consult with your doctor, I suggest you also consider jumping ahead to Chapter Nine, "Overcoming Limitations." Read it right after this chapter and then come back to Chapter Three. I was overwhelmed by the stories of individuals who've managed to overcome their health issues via exercise. Reading those stories and the summaries of issues might motivate you to start a program — with your doctor's approval.

IF YOU QUIT, DON'T GIVE UP

Ever know anyone who smoked and one day just decided to quit and that was the end of it? It isn't likely; there are only estimates of how many times a smoker quits before it becomes permanent but it's at least several times, likely more.

Last spring I congratulated Dave for showing up regularly at our fitness center in SW Florida as I'd not seen him there in the past. He said, "Harry, this is probably the twentieth time I've started an exercise program." The reality is that most people who start an exercise program quit after about six weeks. The question is, how many start up again?

People quit for a variety of reasons: they're discouraged by minimal progress, have company for a week, catch a cold, go away on a trip, whatever. It's easy to say,

"I gave it a try and it didn't work." What about, instead, revisiting the reasons you started a program; did they change? If not, why not give it another try? If you smoked, think back to what it took to quit permanently.

A NEVER GIVE UP STORY

Sandy lives in Easton, NY. I sent the first seven chapters to him at the request of our mutual friend, David. Sandy read them and sent me the following email:

"Thank you, Harry, for all the work you've done. It's a fine book. I've been very active most of my life (running, weights, rode bike to work in NYC, etc.). I began bike racing at age thirty-eight and was training like a madman three hours a day. I've slowed down and now go in and out of fitness. We have a gym in our house — weights, press machine, bikes and rower.

"We also have an active other life, music — I practice several hours a day. Sometimes (often) the psychic energy to work out after playing the piano or organ is lacking. And now, with two to three feet of snow on the ground, fifteen degrees outside and the wind is howling, to hell with it, time for wine!

"But, as I have done always over the years, I just face up to it and start again and again and again. Usually from further behind, but at least we start again. As I read your book I'd anticipate what you "should" have and it would be the next chapter.

"What would I add? I've been thinking about this, reading and training for a long time. You've done a great job. Perhaps I would add just what I said; *sometimes you just have to start over, and maybe later, start over again.* It will be a valuable book for the older person. Good going!"

I'M JUST TOO BUSY

I was listening to NPR recently and heard a discussion of a report I include in the exercise and the brain chapter about the role of aerobic exercise in the growth of the hippocampus. The report included interviews with one of the participants as well as Art Kramer of the University of Illinois, the lead researcher. The hippocampus is a major component of our brain required for the formation of long-term memory and cognitive maps for spatial navigation.

The study involved having one group of participants do an hour of aerobic activity walking on a treadmill three days a week and a control group do stretching, toning and a bit of strength training for the same period of time. Both groups did this for six months.

At the end of the six months the aerobic group showed an increase in the size of their hippocampus while the control group showed a decrease. In addition, the participant interviewed on NPR said that he could tell the difference in his endurance as a direct result of the exercise. In spite of that the interviewed participant elected not to continue the aerobic exercise once the study was over. He said, "I'm just too busy."

If someone said to you, "I'd like to have an hour of your valuable time five days a week. If you'll donate that amount of time to activities that will involve aerobic exercise and strength training, not only will you feel better but you'll live a longer and more active, healthy life. On average you'll gain almost six years of life, but the big deal is that it will be more active and healthy years. Whadda you think?" I hope you'd sign up for this program in a heartbeat! Please, if we ever meet, don't tell me, "I'm just too busy."

BUT GOLF'S MORE FUN

Bill P, a true golf enthusiast, said, "The main difficulty in getting an avid golfer to play less golf and exercise more is that golf is interesting, non-repetitive, challenging, social and competitive. Exercise, for the most part, is not many of those things. If you believe differently, you need to make those points."

Let's compare a few sports:

Cycling — This sport qualifies as interesting, non-repetitive, challenging, social and competitive — in spades. Much of the time we cycle with one or many more people and have lots of social interaction. It's certainly interesting, challenging and as non-repetitive as or more so than golf. We can regularly ride new routes. Competitive — one group I ride with has the KOM — King of the Mountain. When we hit a big hill they go crazy to see who can reach the top first. In Florida we always have a race over a large overpass.

Kayaking — Art loves this sport, does it with his wife and sometimes with a group. This past winter he took a six-day trip in the Everglades with seven friends, camping on beautiful beaches in the Gulf of Mexico. The scenery was gorgeous. There were more large birds flying around than in the Museum of Natural History. In Maine, where he spends the summer, the coastal scenery is beautiful. Kayaking is certainly interesting, non-repetitive, challenging and social. It can be competitive if the paddlers choose to make it so, plus it can support a secondary hobby of wildlife photography.

Running — Those who run would say that their sport of choice also qualifies on all fronts. Many run together and have lots of social interaction. They also find it interesting, challenging and as non-repetitive as they choose. Competitive — Ted, now eighty-one, regularly competes in 5K and even 10K races. Recently Ted was in Quebec City and learned about a 10K race the next morning. He signed up, got up at 5:30 AM to catch the bus to the start, waited two hours, raced — and won in his age group.

Hiking and Walking — All of the above except for competitive. Hiking up mountains is particularly enjoyable and the reward of the views is terrific.

Strength Training and Gym Aerobics — These are generally solo activities and don't pass muster for some of Bill's criteria. They're certainly challenging and competitive — the latter with ourselves, as we like to get stronger. The big ones here are the sense of accomplishment and the feel-good feeling after. This doesn't always happen with golf, particularly after a poor round. As we get older and less fit — particularly if golf is the sole activity — the poor rounds seem to happen with greater frequency.

AN ALTERNATIVE TO ONE GAME

Mark T added the following, addressed to Bill P: "If you gave up one game of golf a week in favor of exercise (the five hours required), you'd be able to play (my estimate) 2,000 more rounds of golf over your lifetime. You might also reach everyman's goal of shooting your age. I heard once that if you can play to a ten handicap at age sixty-five you have a good chance of shooting your age — if you stay in shape. Now that's a lot more of what we enjoy about golf."

ANN'S GROWING UP

Ann is the wife of Sandy, author of the "Never Give Up" story a few pages back. Ann read the chapters I sent to Sandy and added: "This weekend I sat down and read through your upbeat and inspirational book. Of course, I took some time off with my husband Sandy and our two dogs to hike our snow-covered fields, lift weights, row and cycle on our trainers. The dogs slept while we worked out! Thank you not only for your substantial research but also your friendly, colloquial style.

"As a woman who went through parochial schools in the 1950s and early 1960s, I think I'm pretty representative of folks who were taught a great deal about focusing on academics, things of the mind, but ignoring the body. I never took a physical education course, ever. Nor were my parents role models for physical activity. Thank goodness for Jim Fixx, author of *Running*, Nike running shoes and like-minded companions back in the seventies.

"But there are many women my age for whom lifting weights and monitoring their heart rates are things that 'just aren't done.' I applaud your inclusion of osteoporosis/osteopenia, hypertension, etc. as it relates to women. However, I would push the benefits even more to capture women's attention: a greater sense of well-being, the satisfaction that results from being able to lift weights, walk or cycle long distances, increasing self-confidence and pride.

"As we age and retire it's understandable that a sense of loss enters into our lives. Whatever our position had been in the workplace, we not only are no longer there, but we've been replaced. For many women, becoming an older woman is not desirable at all. Gray hair and grandmother status are in opposition to a society focused on youth and energy. This sense of loss can easily become acedia or depression. Once even low-level depression settles in, the motivation to exercise plummets.

"Thank you for a wonderful manuscript."

ONLY FOR THOSE WHO DON'T EXERCISE

Suppose you do not have nor ever have had a serious exercise program. I'm happy that you've been motivated to read this far. Maybe someone gave the book to you and urged you to read it, or maybe you're just curious about what exercise really involves.

If you continue and read the entire book — and I hope you do — you'll be what we'll call an "educated consumer." You'll understand many of the benefits of a serious exercise program as well as some of the consequences of not following one. You can now make an intelligent, educated decision: shall I choose Door A or Door B?

Remember how in business we'd remind ourselves to look at our business, markets and competitors as they are and not how we would like them to be? You now know enough to do that with your body. Patrick Moynihan once said, "We're all entitled to our own opinions but not our own facts." You now have the facts.

If you choose Door B, terrific. It'll require a significant lifestyle change and it won't be easy. But, you will begin to see the benefits quickly. Once you're into a program you'll be glad you made the choice. The longer you do it the easier it gets and the better you'll feel.

If you choose — and it is definitely a choice at this stage — to continue with Door A, you're still ahead of the game as a result of reading this book. Let me explain why.

At some point in the next few years you may experience what we'll call a "catastrophic event." This is when you, your spouse, another relative, a friend or acquaintance — or several of the above — experience a health crisis that may be linked to their lack of fitness. It could be a heart attack, a stroke or, even worse, a death.

Another catalyst could be an annual physical with your doctor that leads to a "come to Jesus discussion" — similar to the hypothetical discussion with my doctor. This is where the doctor's more concerned about you and your future than whether you like him or her. The doctor decides to tell it to you like it is, not as you'd like to think it is. And this time you really listen. It can be something as simple as one day looking in the mirror and realizing that the person you are is not the person you want to be; not even close.

One or more of these events can lead to what we'll call "The Great Awakening." That's when you say to yourself, "If I don't do something I'm going to be in a nursing home or six feet under a lot sooner than I expected. I want to be around to see the grandkids graduate from college and get married. At this rate I may not see them finish high school! I've got to make some changes — maybe I should review that book I read a few years ago by what's his name — where'd I put it?"

The good news is that it's never too late. Earlier is better but later trumps never by a lot. If you can't find the book, no problem; you can purchase another copy, a small investment.

TIM'S GREAT AWAKENING

We all can visualize a roller coaster. That was Tim's exercise program — up, down, even sideways.

When he was on, he was really on — New York Marathon, for example, as well as many others — strength training, running, swimming; he did it all. He understood the value of exercise.

Then he'd get a promotion and start traveling more, wining and dining clients. Exercise would become a thing of the past and sometimes years would go by. Eventually he'd wake up and get back with the program.

In 1998, at the age of fifty-one, he was in A+ shape. But business took priority again and in 2000, he went off the wagon and stayed off. He retired in 2008, relocated to Florida and began doing moderate exercise but nothing like what he'd done in his prime. In October 2009, he was in Chicago visiting his daughter and went to her gym to work out. When he got on the treadmill he felt a twinge in his chest; not pain, just discomfort. The same thing happened a few days later. He went back to Florida and thought no more of it.

Fortunately, he'd made an appointment for a physical exam months earlier with a new doctor. If he hadn't he wouldn't have taken action. An EKG confirmed that he had a serious problem. The next day a cardiologist saw him, did additional tests and put him in the hospital — immediately. Two days later he had open heart surgery. It turned out he had ninety-eight percent blockage in two of his arteries.

He came out of the hospital a new man. He began walking and in four weeks was at the stage in recovery where most are in three months. The physical therapist discharged him way ahead of others based on his progress and commitment.

He's again in A+ shape. He does five hours of aerobics work weekly, three days a week of strength training and three days of swimming. He does aerobics at sixty percent to seventy-five percent of his maximum heart rate and his strength training is to fatigue. His wife calls him a "gym rat." He's lost over thirty pounds. Tim said, "It isn't often you get a mulligan in your life and it was an easy decision to take full advantage of it." (If you're not a golfer, a mulligan is a second chance.)

PEGGY'S STORY

Peggy lives in my community in SW Florida. In 2003, the Fitness Center staff asked her if she would like to work with them on a special assignment. She said yes — after all, how could she not want to improve her physical condition with the help of these pros? She told this story:

"How many times have you or one of your neighbors said, 'We're so lucky to live here?' It's so true, and the Fitness Center is one of the reasons. I feel especially lucky because I spent much of this summer at the center on a regular basis. The staff there asked if I'd like to be a test case for the eight fitness professionals to assess.

"From May to October, I worked with each of the trainers on an individual basis. A personalized nutrition program was also set up after I'd completed an in-depth food questionnaire about my eating habits. I learned the value of consuming fewer calories, eating healthier foods, eating reasonably sized portions, excellent supplements and, the best part, five or six meals a day.

"All of the fitness professionals, with their clipboards in hand, analyzed my physical condition. In the first assessment in May I felt like I was under a microscope: I stretched, walked, bent and stood on one leg and then the other — with eyes open and eyes closed. These professionals were thorough!

"Each of the professionals designed workouts based on my situation. I learned about resistance training and weights and the benefits of working opposing muscle groups. We worked on what the trainers called the 'big three': aerobics, stretching and strength training.

"I'm happy to report that quantifiable results show I've lost weight, body fat and inches. I lost ten pounds and seven percent of body fat. The Fitness Center has become a habit for me. I realize that getting there regularly is a lifestyle change. Even with the busy schedules that we all have, it's possible to carve out time to exercise. Working out truly does make me feel better.

"Fitness professionals can make all the difference. If your budget and/or schedule only allow an occasional session with a pro, that's all it takes to jump-start a targeted and safe routine. A trainer can keep you on track by modifying your workout. They're pros at adding variety (eliminating any excuses about getting bored) and addressing any changes in your physical condition.

"Eating well is also a lifestyle change; a good nutritious program doesn't have to be a diet. The scale hasn't surged. It seems that exercise and eating really do go hand in hand."

Eight years later:

"Do I still work out at the Fitness Center on a regular basis? The honest answer is no, not as frequently. But I'm still hooked and work out at least a few times every week. I've maintained the weight loss (though haven't checked the body fat lately!), and I still work hard at keeping the calories in check. Being active and working at keeping fit are definite habits for me — thanks to an excellent fitness program started years ago."

I'VE GOT A PLAN

Bill Y read this chapter and wrote the following:

"An area you discuss that rings with me is planning. I personally find that when I plan the day it's easy to add an hour or more of exercise. When I do that, I generally honor the process by doing it. Somehow, when I put exercise into the schedule exercise has been raised to another level — a level that means I need to do it, just like going to the bank, broker, etc. When I don't take the time to build a schedule I find all kinds of ways to waste the time. I become lethargic. It becomes too easy to say, 'I'll do it tomorrow.'

"Unfortunately, I think that many retired people interpret retirement to mean no schedules. Wrong. It only means I don't need to follow someone else's schedule. I still need to build my own if I want a sense of well-being and purpose. None of us do anything without some kind of planning. I think of the time that it takes to arrange a golf tee time. I have to look at

> the calendar, decide when to request a time, make the call or use the web, etc.; all planning."

TRY THIS

Let's say that you're thinking about going to your fitness center tomorrow morning. Notice I said "thinking about it" versus "you're going to go." That way of thinking applies to all of us at various times. How can you move to a commitment?

One idea is to prepare the night before. Put the clothes you need to wear to the gym out in prominent view so that the logical step is to put them on the next morning. That makes the next logical step to just go. Little steps like this can be the tipping point.

TIMING'S EVERYTHING

Behavioral economics has become a popular field in recent years. One area of research has shown that we tend to make better decisions about the future for ourselves than we do for the present.

Suppose someone is twenty pounds heavier than they should be, and I said to that person, "Would you be willing to make a commitment to lose twenty pounds in six months, beginning six months from now?" The likely response is yes.

We'll change the rules a bit. How about committing to start losing twenty pounds beginning tomorrow? Well, now that's different. That means that they have to take action now, not at some future date. They're willing to commit to begin exercising or eating a healthy diet in the future, but right now — they're not sure about that.

The reality is that if you're going to change your life now's the time, not some future date.

WHAT'S THE END GAME?

What would you like to be doing when you're eighty? Travel, for example, or enjoying sports activities such as golf, tennis or cycling? You certainly would like to be able to do vigorous walking. Spending time with grandkids is generally a high priority. Wouldn't it be nice if you could do some physical activities with them?

Now to the hard part; what do you need to do so that you can do those things? And how does it differ from what you're doing now?

Say you're currently sixty-five; the actuary guys say that, on average, you'll live to about eighty-three years. You have a fifty percent chance of living beyond that and a twenty-five percent chance that you'll live five years longer. On top of that, one in twenty will live to his or her early nineties.

What do you want those years to look like? Being healthy and active sure trumps unhealthy and inactive by a long shot. While there's no magic pill that you can take at age seventy-eight or any age that will make up for inaction before then, you can improve your health by exercising.

The biggest advance in modern medicine is not a new drug. Rather, it's the knowledge that what we can do to manage our lives can help us to live longer and happier. The most important changes are lifestyle (activity and exercise) and diet. We're all going to die, but we can delay the inevitable by quite a bit and gain more enjoyment between now and then. The goal is to lead an active, healthy life, not just be alive.

Nike got it right: "Just Do It." Get out there — whether it's with your wife, kids, grandkids and friends or a whole new group of people you'll learn to socialize with, or even by yourself — and make that effort that will pay off big-time. In a bacon and egg breakfast the chicken is involved, but the pig is committed. When it comes to exercise, we need to be involved and committed.

IT GETS TO BE FUN

Ever hear a golfer say, "I've got to go play golf again today"? One of my golf addict friends said years ago, "I'd rather play golf than eat." And he liked to eat.

Many of my cycling friends feel the same way about their sport. Those who work can't wait for Saturday and Sunday when they can go for long rides, and in the summer, many get up to ride before work. They know it's good for their bodies and minds, which may have been the original reason, but it gets to be an enormous amount of fun. It's just as much fun to them as golf is to golf enthusiasts.

Others look forward to their trips to their gym. They enjoy the challenge of aerobic and strength training. Imagine the feeling of satisfaction of increasing the weight used for a specific exercise from thirty to forty pounds over several months.

This can happen to you — if you give it enough time.

Anahad O'Connor wrote an article in *The New York Times* in 2011 about centenarians. He quoted from research done by Dr. Nir Barzilai, director of the Institute for Aging Research at Einstein College of Medicine. He thinks that both diet and exercise are crucial, particularly if you don't have parents, aunts or uncles who've lived a long life.

He said; "If you listen to what your doctor is telling you and watch your weight, drink a glass of wine a day, exercise, avoid smoking and treat any conditions like high blood pressure, you're likely to get to over the age of eighty."

CHECK OUT YOUR LIFE

The American Heart Association has a questionnaire, My Life Check — Life's Simple 7 — the website is mylifecheck.Heart.org. Take a few minutes to complete it to get a measure of where you are today. It's a good step as you begin reading this book.

WAITING FOR SUPERMAN

The title above comes from a film documentary on the status of education in America. It's from Geoffrey Canada, founder of Harlem Children's Zone, a highly successful charter school in New York. His school has properly received lots of publicity.

Canada grew up in Harlem in a very poor family. As a young child he thought that everything would be okay because Superman would save him. He truly believed in Superman.

He was devastated when he learned that Superman didn't really exist. He didn't know who was going to save him so he ended up saving himself. His story, and the story of his school, is very inspirational.

You, of course, have always known that Superman isn't real. And at least for your adult life you've known that the only person who can save you is yourself. What are YOU waiting for? The decisions you make now will determine whether you lead an active, healthy life over the next twenty or more years.

A POOL PLAYER'S ADVICE

Mark T, a serious pool player, said:

"Pool players say, 'Experience is what you get immediately following the time in which you needed it.' Hopefully that won't be the epitaph for those who did not heed the preaching of this book."

LET'S REVIEW

- Investing an hour a day in your health can pay huge dividends in the quality of your life and the number of years of quality living.

- Almost everyone quits exercise at some point. The key to success is starting over, and sometimes, starting over again. Never give up.

- Reading this book is one step. It may take a Great Awakening to get you going.

- Think about what you'd like to be doing ten, fifteen and twenty years from now. Then think about what you need to do — now — to make that happen.

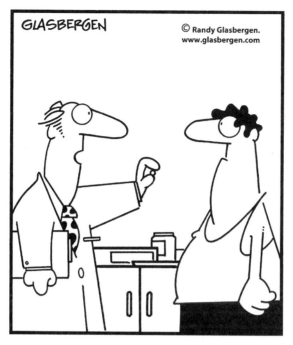

"To prevent a heart attack, take one aspirin every day. Take it out for a run, then take it to the gym, then take it for a bike ride..."

CHAPTER THREE — GETTING GOING AND KEEPING GOING

"The person determined to achieve maximum success learns the principle that progress is made one step at a time. A house is built one brick at a time. Football games are won a play at a time. Every big accomplishment is a series of little accomplishments."

—David Joseph Schwartz, PH.D., author of The Magic of Thinking Big

HERE'S WHAT'S COMING

- Intrinsic and extrinsic motivation — what's the difference?
- Is the Curve of Pistophenes a normal part of learning something new?
- Why is finding an action trigger a big deal?
- Why is writing goals down so important?
- How do you make a habit out of doing the right stuff?
- What's a BHAG?

I'M JUST NOT MOTIVATED

Beginning in 1919, a group of New York intellectuals called the Algonquin Round Table gathered at the Algonquin Hotel regularly. One day a member of the group, Dorothy Parker, was challenged to use the word "horticulture" in a sentence. Within seconds she said, "You can lead a horticulture but you cannot make her think."

I thought of that when a friend who'd expressed interest in starting a training program balked when I brought it up later. When he'd mentioned it several weeks earlier I bought a favorite fitness book for him that I thought might help get him started, but he didn't read it.

We were at a party and, after a few glasses of wine, he listened to my encouraging (?) words and said, "I know you're trying to help me, but I'm just not motivated." What did I do? I changed the subject. I learned a lesson that I seem to have to learn over and over: *nobody, but nobody, is going to make a lifestyle change until they are good and ready.* In order to start exercising, change eating habits, quit smoking, quit or reduce drinking or break a drug addiction — *motivation has to come from within.*

INTRINSIC OR EXTRINSIC?

Whether you stick with an exercise program is influenced greatly by whether it's an intrinsic or extrinsic behavior. If it begins as extrinsic can you, over time, convert it to intrinsic?

We'll define **intrinsic behaviors** as those we do because we enjoy the activities and we may also be proficient at them. A classic example is golf; I've never heard a golfer say, "I've got to play golf today." Even those who have a high handicap enjoy it as an intellectual, physical and social activity. Many of all ability levels are passionate about the game and play as frequently as they can. The only thing it takes to motivate them is having a tee time and some friends to play with. Other sports can be in this category also, depending upon the individual. Many runners, tennis players and cyclists have a similar view of their sport.

Extrinsic behaviors are those we do in order to obtain benefits from the activity. Virtually everyone who goes on a diet is implementing an extrinsic behavior. They want to lose weight and thereby improve their health. Does anyone on a diet say, "I sure enjoy being on this diet"? I suspect very few do. If they choose to make a lifestyle change involving healthy eating versus going on a diet, then it can be a different story.

Another way to think of these is that intrinsic behaviors are ones we want to do and extrinsic are ones we should or need to do. Clearly the probability of maintaining an exercise program is higher if it's intrinsic. But an extrinsic program is okay if we can find a way to convert at least the motivational element from extrinsic to intrinsic.

Let's look at the case of aerobic exercise. Do some people really look forward to doing an exercise that gets their heart pumping? Sure they do. Many walkers thoroughly enjoy it, both for the social engagement as well as the physical activity. The same can be said for runners, cyclists, kayakers and those in other aerobic sports. This doesn't mean, of course, that they felt that way the first few times. Their enjoyment increased over time, along with their ability.

Does anyone ever say, "I get to go to the gym today"? Yes, but not with the same frequency as those who play golf or enjoy some other sports. It takes more time to get to the point of feeling that way. Some who go regularly may never get to that point — but they still go.

RICK'S MOTIVATION

Rick meets me at my garage on the days we cycle in SW Florida. Recently on a cold, windy morning I explained the definitions of intrinsic and extrinsic behaviors and asked him where cycling rated for him. Rick thought for a minute and said:

"It depends; when I get up on a day like today, read forty-six degrees on the thermometer and then listen to the Weather Channel forecast of fifteen miles per hour wind out of the north, it's definitely extrinsic. But when we've done our hard ride north into the wind and turn south with the wind at our backs and then stop for coffee — by that time it's intrinsic. It's always intrinsic the last few miles and when I get home I'm always glad I did it."

A FORMULA FOR SUCCESS

Consider this formula: EB + F + T > IB: *Extrinsic behavior plus frequency plus time may lead to intrinsic behavior.*

Remember when you were young and were introduced to a new athletic activity — riding a bicycle, playing tennis, baseball, basketball, whatever — were any of these immediately an intrinsic behavior? It's not likely; you may have had the potential to perform but you lacked experience. You needed to practice and have time to learn before it could become intrinsic.

Halyna said, "I think for many children learning a new sport at a young age is fun and a game, so they tend to be enthusiastic about it, at least at the outset. I think of our grandkids, who eagerly want to learn and get better at various ball games."

As adults we tend to gravitate to those activities that have become intrinsic. We know some others are definitely good for us but are extrinsic — aerobic activity, strength training and healthy eating come to mind — but many of us don't take the time for our interest in these activities to become intrinsic. It's no surprise that we tend to give up on extrinsic behaviors at a much more rapid rate than we do intrinsic ones.

Once we've made the decision that a specific activity will have a positive effect on our ability to lead an active, healthy life, we need to make a commitment to stick with it. It may ultimately be a matter of discipline — for many of us strength training may never become intrinsic, for example, but we'll always feel better for having done it.

LET'S GET REAL

Other than sex, what activity can we name that was immediately intrinsic? Even sex doesn't totally qualify; while it certainly was immediately enjoyable we weren't necessarily proficient. It was definitely something you wanted to do again, and you didn't say to yourself, "Oh, I have to have sex today." Must we become highly proficient at an activity for it to become enjoyable and therefore intrinsic? Of course not. Hopefully we became more proficient at sex after we made a commitment to stick with it.

Years ago I read a speech someone gave to a group of life insurance salespeople. The message that stuck with me was that those who were the most successful were those who were willing to do the things in the job that were the least fun, like making cold calls on prospects. They did the tasks that were less fun because they knew they were important to their success. It's unlikely that making cold calls ever became an intrinsic behavior.

What drives someone to overcome their discomfort or lack of motivation to implement a beneficial behavior? Maybe it's their vision of success and its rewards. Having a picture of the "end product" and keeping it in mind can be motivational. We need to do that with our exercise program.

AL ROKER

"The Today Show" interviewed Al Roker, one of the stars on their show, about his weight loss over the last ten years. He told the story of visiting his father when they both knew his father was dying. His father extracted a promise from Al that he would deal with his weight problem; he was 340 pounds at the time. His father said he wanted Al to be around to see his kids grow up, particularly since their grandfather would not be.

Al had bariatric surgery in 2002, and now weighs in at about 200 pounds. He exercises regularly, doing aerobics and strength training in a gym. He said that he's had some relapses and has to continue to fight for control. Al said several times: "The motivation has to come from within."

FEAR AS MOTIVATION

Chris is one of my SW Florida cycling buddies; we ride three times a week. Over forty years ago, when he was twenty-seven, Chris had a physical exam. He can't remember his diastolic blood pressure but his systolic was 190.

Systolic is the peak pressure in the arteries at the moment the heart muscle is contracting and **diastolic** is the minimum pressure during the period between beats when the heart is resting. The doctor told him he should put him in the hospital. He also said, "Either you start exercising and lose forty pounds or you'll be dead in two years. You better make out a will."

Fear can be a strong motivator for some of us. Chris got the message, joined a gym, stopped eating junk, got in shape and stayed that way. When he turned sixty he decided to do something hard. He signed up with a cycling company and rode with a group from Oregon to New Hampshire.

Rain or shine, up and down mountains, into strong headwinds, they rode every day for nearly two months.

More recently he and some pals cycled the Going to the Sun Road in Glacier National Park, Montana — a 3,500-foot climb in nine miles. They then cycled from Banff to Jasper, Canada, a 150-mile ride up the Icefields Parkway in the Canadian Rockies with lots of climbing alongside what he described as incredibly beautiful glaciers.

He also goes to the gym regularly and does serious strength training, not just moving a few light weights. Chris is clearly motivated. Cycling has become an intrinsic behavior.

The story about Chris is of a man who took his fitness training and exercises *very* seriously. I don't want you to come away with the idea that the level of fitness he's attained needs to be, or even should be, your goal. Rather, I want you to know that there are different kinds of fitness activities and a fitness level that is right for you. It will be up to you to find that level, but one thing is really not optional: you have to become committed and stay that way. Only a steadfast commitment that will carry you over the occasional bumps along the way will bring you the satisfaction and sense of well-being that you want and should have.

Do you want to play golf through your seventies and beyond, stay out of the hospital, avoid high blood pressure, type 2 diabetes, joint replacements and a myriad of other ailments that come with age and lack of physical fitness? You can do it.

Is it easy? Can you do it without changing your lifestyle? Not likely. Initially it's work and it takes time before it gets to be fun. As a friend said, "There're only two times to exercise; when you feel like it and when you don't."

EVER FUN?

Halyna added, "This comment makes it sound like it's never gonna be fun — will always be work. And maybe that's OK, even if we realize that strength training, for example, may always be extrinsic, that doesn't mean we won't be motivated to do it, since we know the end result will give us the benefits we're looking for. Kind of like going to work — even when you love your job/career, there are times when you don't want to go but have to go, and the end result/benefit is that paycheck that we want, which will allow us the lifestyle we want."

Years ago, in a company I worked for, we hired Jim fresh out of the Marine Corps. A two-tour Vietnam veteran who was awarded two Bronze Stars and attained the rank of captain, Jim spent his entire career with that company and retired a few years ago. I recall his saying when he joined the company, "The hardest part of this job is starting over as the new man again."

When you start a training program, you're the new man (or woman) again. You're in an unfamiliar environment, around different people and may have a general feeling of discomfort, like, "What am I doing here?" It takes some determination to get past this.

What should you do? Join a gym and sign up for some sessions with a trainer who will develop a program of aerobic and strength training based on your current fitness level. Begin easy and work up after your muscles have adapted to the new stresses you're placing on them. Too hard, too soon equal sore muscles, discouragement and a strong desire to quit. I'll provide more information about trainers and what to do if you don't choose to use one in later chapters. And the great news is that it's never too late. Residents of nursing homes in their nineties have benefited significantly from aerobic and strength training within a few months.

What can we do for friends who need to make a change but aren't motivated? We can listen and, if they ever decide on their own, we can provide support and encouragement.

THE CURVE OF PISTOPHENES

In the mid-1980s, I met Neil Rackham, a native of the U.K., who developed a terrific sales training program, "Spin Selling." He also wrote a bestselling book on the topic.

Neil introduced the work of the "famous Greek philosopher," Pistophenes, who originated the Learning Curve. The curve is steep as we try to implement new ideas and techniques and then levels off once we master them. In the process we may get a bit "pissed off" at the steepness of our learning curve. Neil labeled this frustration with the name of an imaginary Greek philosopher.

The Curve of Pistophenes is normal in developing and implementing a fitness program. It takes awhile to master the right way of doing things. We don't see results immediately; that takes a few weeks or months. We may be sore since we're using muscles that haven't been really utilized for decades in some cases. What do we expect those muscles to do other than complain? We have to work our way through the curve. And as we progress, the curve will become less steep. We have to stick to it.

DAMN . . .

Vicki wrote: "It's also good to include that it's not always fun because it's hard at times, but I can't say I've ever walked away from a workout saying, 'Damn, I wish I hadn't done that.' The same with motivation...I joke (and am also serious) with my husband Dan using the same comment with regard to sex; sex is like going to the gym — I don't always feel like it but I never walk away saying, 'Damn!'"

Halyna added: "Truer words have rarely been spoken (on both counts)... the other day Bill and I dragged ourselves to the gym, but came out saying to each other — sure glad we went."

EVERY DAY, IN EVERY WAY, I'M GETTING BETTER AND BETTER

Sound appealing? A Frenchman named Émile Coué introduced this idea in the early 1900s. A psychologist and pharmacist, he would tell some recipients of his medicines that the medicines would produce fantastic results, and they would. He would tell others nothing and the results were not nearly as good.

Coué observed that the main obstacle to autosuggestion, or positive thinking, was willpower. The patient must not let his will impose views on positive ideas. Everything must be done to ensure that the positive idea is consciously accepted by the patient.

Coué's work served as the foundation for many successful books: *The Power of Positive Thinking* by Norman Vincent Peale; *Think and Grow Rich* by Napoleon Hill; *The Magic of Thinking Big* by David Schwartz; and many others. A modern-day author on positive thinking is Tony Robbins. Gazillions of books have been sold based on this idea.

So what does this have to do with exercise? What we have to do is come up with ways to think positively and get past the temptation to quit, using ideas like the action trigger discussed in the next section. Given time it becomes a habit. The results start feeding the habit and away we go.

Scott read this and said about his own exercise journey; "I realized the value of visualization and positive programming; interrupting negative self doubt with an affirmation that I was in the process of achieving/becoming what I wanted."

Apply Harry's mantra: *"Every day that I exercise, I get better and I feel better."*

When you don't really want to do it, think of Pistophenes and just go do it. Remember Harry's mantra and what Vicki said: "Afterwards, exercise or sex, I never regret it."

FIND AN ACTION TRIGGER

I've been reading an interesting book — *Switch: How to Change Things When Change Is Hard* by Chip and Dan Heath.

As the title says, change is frequently hard. Changing from a person who does little or no exercise to one who does it regularly certainly falls into the hard category. It might be below quitting smoking but not very far below. Like smoking, only one person makes the decision.

The Heaths write about the work of two psychologists, Peter Gollwitzer and Veronika Brandstatter, who've been pioneers in the research on action triggers — the idea of tying a specific action, like exercise, to a certain situation.

Example: "I'm going to walk a minimum of one mile a day beginning Wednesday morning after breakfast, before I do anything else. I will do this every day going forward, right after breakfast." *This is a specific plan;*

the walk is triggered by the eating of breakfast.

A poor example: "I should get some exercise; maybe I'll go over to the bookstore next week, pick up an exercise book to read." There is no specific action trigger here.

The researchers tested a group of patients recovering from hip or knee replacement. Those who were asked to set action triggers, such as writing down when and where they planned to walk, had a dramatic increase in their rate of recovery versus those who didn't have a plan. They were bathing themselves without assistance in three weeks versus seven weeks for the others. Heath and Heath said that an analysis of 8,155 participants across eighty-five studies found that the typical person who set an action trigger did better than seventy-four percent of those who didn't set one.

Find an action trigger. Tie your involvement in exercise to a specific, everyday situation.

PAINT A PICTURE — IN YOUR MIND

Chip and Dan Heath tell another story about a Teach for America teacher in Atlanta who was assigned to a class of first graders. Most of them had not attended kindergarten, so she was their first teacher. None were at the level where they needed to be.

She confidently announced at the beginning of the year that "you're going to be third graders by the end of the school year." She meant, of course, in terms of their skill level. She also called her students "scholars" and asked them to address each other that way.

Their test scores had reached second-grade level by the spring, so Crystal threw a graduation party. She changed the way they addressed each other from "scholars" to "second graders". By the end of the year ninety percent of the students were reading at or above a third-grade level.

She painted a picture in their minds of what they could be and the students responded with enthusiasm. You can, too.

THE POWER OF THE WRITTEN WORD

Here's a suggestion that all of us will benefit from: *Write it down.*

You may say, "Write down what?" Why not begin with your goals. Are you committing to an aerobics and strength-training program in order to improve your fitness and health? How about healthy eating more often? If you happen to be overweight, the combination of these three will work magic on your body. Write long sentences, use bullet points or a combination of the two — whatever works for you. Writing it down will help solidify your commitment. Sharing it with your spouse or significant other and friends also helps.

Open a file folder on your computer entitled, "Commitment," or use a notepad. Write down what you are willing to commit to now and revisit it regularly to see if you're living up to your commitment. You may revise it in a few months, and are more likely to add more if you've stuck with the program.

Later I'll talk about the importance of keeping records of your exercise program. This is a powerful complement to your commitment and will fit nicely in the same computer folder.

WORKING TOGETHER

David said: "In order to be successful your spouse has to be on board, especially if you're not yet retired and you have family obligations. In order to have stress-free exercising, discuss your intentions ahead of time. Example: 'I plan on going for a ride at 7 AM and I'll be back by nine.' If that doesn't work ask your 'better half' what the most convenient time for you to exercise is. Be flexible. If you want to go for a three- to four-hour bike ride but you sense that would cause some stress in the house, change it to one to two hours and do a longer ride another day.

"You retired guys have all the breaks!"

SETTING GOALS

I think there's a natural reluctance to write down health and fitness goals. I have no scientific data to back this up, just personal intuition.

Why is this? A factor for those who are new to exercise may be that if they write down goals and don't achieve them, they don't feel very good about themselves. On the other hand, if they start exercising and fall short of their unwritten expectations, somehow it's not so bad. The thought process may be something like, "I never really said I was going to lose twenty pounds in six months, so the fact that I only lost ten is OK."

The act of writing down your goals and even sharing them with your spouse and friends will definitely increase your chances of sticking with them and achieving them. Sharing makes them a commitment versus an idea, a big difference.

Many of us at various times in our lives had to prepare a budget for business. We had to write down what we were going to spend in various categories and also indicate some performance goals. Those goals might be revenue, production numbers, whatever. We were making a commitment of what we were going to do over the next twelve months.

What if we spent the money but fell short of the performance goal? That, of course, was a problem. What many of us would do, if we were falling short on the performance side, was figure out how to ratchet down some of the expenses so that we could come closer or maybe even achieve our bottom-line target.

Let's apply that to setting health and fitness goals. Suppose one of our goals was to lose twenty pounds in six months by a combination of healthy eating and increased exercise. Let's say the exercise target was to walk two miles five days a week, beginning at a pace of three miles per hour and increasing to four miles an hour over six months. What if we found after a few months that we were walking four days instead of five and struggling to get above three and a half miles per hour?

If we're walking less and slower, we're burning fewer calories, making the goal of twenty pounds of weight loss less likely. One option, just like lowering the expenses, would be to reduce our caloric intake so that we can achieve the twenty-pound goal. We can achieve one goal, come close on the second and feel good about ourselves.

Are our chances better of hitting at least one target if we have a written set of goals? Yes, they are. And, it'll be a lot easier to walk four miles an hour versus three or three and a half once we've dropped those twenty pounds.

BIG HAIRY AUDACIOUS GOALS

My son Michael is a training and development consultant. One of the programs he delivers is titled "Remember the Future." He has employees of a company break into small groups and write down what Jim Collins in his book, *Good to Great*, calls "Big Hairy Audacious Goals" (BHAG). In this exercise they assume they've achieved some incredible goal and then work together on the steps it took to get there. The idea is to get them to think big.

I recently participated in a program with a dozen members of our fitness center in SW Florida. We had an assessment at the beginning of the program of weight, waist, blood pressure, etc. and will do the same at the end of eight weeks. We've committed to keeping records of our exercise and eating on a daily basis.

During the kickoff session we were asked to talk about our goals for the eight-week period. Most centered on a loss of ten or more pounds. Mike, the leader, asked us to think deeper — what was the real goal behind the surface goal? One member, for example, wanted to look good at his granddaughter's wedding in June.

My surface goal was to lose five pounds and add some muscle mass, but Mike got me thinking about what my real goal was. After some thought I came up with it: *I want to be able to do what I'm doing today seventeen years from now, when I'm ninety.*

Every year my son and I plus several friends do a Bucks County Birthday Ride in September. The objective is to cycle my age in miles in the rolling hills of Bucks County, PA. Last year four of us did seventy-three miles. One year we had friends from San Francisco, Las Vegas, Bucks County and the United Kingdom. We started this event when I turned seventy.

I want to do eighty miles at eighty years and ninety miles at ninety years. I think that qualifies as a BHAG. It means I have to think today about what I'm doing to take care of myself for the future. That means developing a plan, setting goals, evaluating progress and, if necessary, re-planning and re-establishing goals. This is a dynamic exercise, but it starts with goal setting and planning.

If my lifestyle includes drinking too much wine, for example, it's likely that the cumulative effect of that extra wine will cost me dearly ten or more years from now. The same can be said for eating too much ice cream, which I love. Is it worth it? How does this component of my lifestyle interact with my BHAG?

An occasional extra glass or two of wine is okay. Being too rigid is not only boring but also tough to maintain. I'll have ice cream from time to time, but much more often I'll choose nonfat yogurt.

Think about what a BHAG would be for you. Then think about what you need to do to get there.

GOAL SUMMARY

- If you're new to this, set a date to get started — and stick with it.
- Write down your goals and review what you wrote at least weekly.
- Share your goals with your significant other and one or more friends. Ask for their support.
- Have a plan on how to achieve that goal. Make a daily appointment to exercise — put it on your calendar — and stick with it.
- Find an action trigger for daily motivation.
- Keep records daily of what you eat and the exercise you do.
- Celebrate success. Reward yourself in some way.
- Be sure your goals are not too hard and therefore unrealistic, or too easy to achieve. Do a reality check periodically.
- Have a set of goals for twelve months, then another set for another twelve months.
- Once you're into it, set a BHAG. It's fun to think about what will qualify.
- There's a goal-setting template in the Appendix. See if it works for you as a model.

THE SECRET SAUCE

Mark read the first seven chapters in draft and wrote the following when he read the above section:

"I think that health, as many others things, must be managed by the person. I also believe strongly that you cannot manage what you cannot measure. Getting a set of metrics in place that will track progress is important. This can relate to repetitions, weights, running pace, number of drinks a week, body mass index, miles per hour on treadmill, time to run a mile or bike ten, etc. This kind of scorecard will help you track weekly and/or monthly progress, much like the monthly income statement and balance sheet in business.

"I'm also a huge fan of the BHAG — for me, this is the ability to someday shoot my age in golf. BHAG's should be attainable and they shouldn't be so far into the future that you can get away with not doing something now. I've heard that one's ability to shoot one's age in golf dramatically improves if you can have a single digit handicap at the age of sixty-five. This isn't so far ahead for me that I can put off the hard work. In the meantime I know that getting to a six handicap or less at sixty-two is important. I'm now fifty-nine.

"If you want to get somewhere you've got to know where it is you're trying to go. You need a set of metrics that will help you evaluate progress and should have a dedication to measuring them. As I think about this book what becomes clear to me is that I have some ability to control my life as I age.

"The overriding goal for everyone who will take action based on this book is to live a productive and active life right up till the end. You've given enough proof points to help the reader see that it's possible. You've explained well that one can, through exercise, help avoid mental deterioration. You've also explained that keeping fit can mean many additional years of enjoying the grandkids and playing golf. You've given many helpful tips on how we can develop ourselves in order to avoid the thing we all dread — incapacity.

"You're trying to create a method through which one can begin the journey toward continuing the joy one has had thus far for the remainder of this time on earth. It's a most important chapter. Without it you could get many people to 'enjoy' the book but few to actually do something about it — because it's difficult to start.

"Now you're going to give them the 'secret sauce.' You've enlivened the dream of productivity into the later years of life and now you can get them to begin to live that dream. The keys you are attempting to get across are the power of goals that drive strategy. How about beating your grandson in a race when he's ten years old? Select the short-term measurement of some set of metrics that will keep you posted on progress.

"In the book you give, appropriately so, wide latitude to strategy. One can bike, run, play tennis, swim, etc. This is very good but also can create a lack of focus for an individual — this chapter demands that one set out their particular program — every day lost makes it that much less certain that the productivity sought will be achieved.

"Getting as specific as possible in helping the reader to establish a measurement system and clarify their goals can be the action point that makes this book important, not just interesting data.

"You should know that I've taken the message to heart. Now I must get off to the gym. On Saturday I leave for a skiing vacation with our family. I'm certain that I will outski my four-year-old grandson this year — but what about when I'm seventy and he's fifteen? I think I have every right to believe that I will be able to ski with him (run for run) at that time too — thanks to you."

REGINA AND CORT: TWO HUNDRED AND ONE

Regina knew things were out of control when she found it took too much effort to get up from the chair at her desk to get something — she started asking Cort to do it for her. She was five feet two inches tall and tipped the scales at 276 pounds — four and a half pounds per inch of height. That was March 2008. She and Cort are in their early sixties.

Cort was going away for a month and she made up her mind that it was time to change. Regina had her Great Awakening. She began having Instant Breakfast twice a day and then a normal dinner. She had no dessert of any kind, always her Achilles' heel. She said nothing to Cort.

She started exercising by walking on the treadmill. As she said, "I began some exercise: initially one-quarter mile, then one-half mile and by the end of two weeks one mile. By the end of the first month I was walking three miles a day on the treadmill."

Regina went from walking a quarter of a mile to three miles — in a month. Think about what a huge change that is. This is for a woman five feet two inches tall, 276 pounds.

Regina and Cort don't get an A+ for communication. It turns out Cort had the same idea but didn't tell Regina. During the month Cort was away Regina dropped twenty pounds — and Cort dropped ten. Then they started working together on exercise and eating habits.

By September 2009, Regina reached her goal weight of 125 pounds and now stays between 118 and 124. Cort dropped from 245 to 195 and stays there, plus or minus a couple of pounds. Let's do the math: 276–125 = 151; 245–195 = 50; 151 + 50 = 201. What a formula.

Regina said: "We weigh in every day — we record our weight on a chart. We record the number of steps our pedometers read. We record our activity (walking on a carriage road in Maine, on a treadmill, etc.) and we record our indiscretions such as a cookie extravaganza, ice cream or what-have-you."

Recording activity can provide motivation. If you keep track, who wants to write down "Today I did nothing"?

REWARD YOURSELF

You can come up with ways that you can give yourself a reward for living up to your exercise commitment. If you go to the gym, for a long walk, a bike ride, you may choose to have an ice cream cone that night after dinner. You've earned it.

At work we used to do the hard projects first at the beginning of the day and then tackle the easier problems. You can apply the same principle to doing your exercise first and then do things that are, for the moment at least, more intrinsic.

In the action trigger mentioned above, consider using breakfast as a reward. If you enjoy eating breakfast, then you could say to yourself, "Beginning this coming Wednesday I'm going to walk one mile a day before breakfast." By using the trigger as a reward for sticking to your plan, the trigger becomes even more powerful.

With a little creativity you can easily design an action trigger and reward that work for you.

WHAT'S A HABIT?

A habit is simply an implementation of behavioral autopilot. We have lots of habits we've formed over the years, intentional or not, good or bad. We buckle our seatbelt before starting the car, put our leg in our right pants leg first versus the left and brush our teeth in exactly the same way every day. Implementing a new habit is simply a matter of allocating enough time for it to happen.

Vince Lombardi said, "Once you learn to quit, it becomes a habit." That's one habit you don't want to develop.

I HAVE A DREAM

These are likely among the best-known words in the English language as a result of Martin Luther King's speech delivered on August 28, 1963, at the Lincoln Memorial in Washington, D.C. We should have a dream also. Paint a picture in your mind of what will be different six months from now as a result of your action plan. Then write it down — and share it with others.

SELF-EFFICACY AND EXERCISE

Psychologist Albert Bandura defined self-efficacy as the belief in one's ability to succeed in specific situations. The stronger a person's sense of self-efficacy, the more likely he or she will view that they can master a new task, even a difficult one.

Self-efficacy is situation-specific; someone who believes they can lose twenty pounds by exercise and healthy eating won't necessarily think they can climb Mt. Everest. As Clint Eastwood said, "A man's got to know his limitations."

The more successful someone has been in the past at accomplishing goals, the more likely they will have a high sense of self-efficacy; a belief that they can accomplish a new goal. Also, research has shown that participation in a group working to achieve the same or a similar goal increases the likelihood of success. Socializing and having fun helps.

Whether you're thinking about starting an exercise program or find yourself struggling to stay motivated in one, try thinking back to something you've done in your life that was really hard, where you ultimately succeeded. How does this compare to that?

Many decades ago I decided to quit smoking. Not try to quit, which I'd done several times before, but really quit for good. The big difference was that I said to myself, family and friends, "I'm quitting smoking as of right now." That was over forty years ago. Making a firm decision to quit made it much easier.

Think ahead to how much better you'll feel about yourself once you've stuck with a program and seen the results in energy, mood and health. You'll have even more self-efficacy to tackle the next big task.

Recently I got up on a rainy day, a day that was supposed to be a cycling day with a friend in Bucks County, PA. Since cycling was out I knew I should go to the gym, but my body felt stiff and I had a mild pain in one knee. I was beginning to think up reasons why I wouldn't go when I decided to reread portions of this chapter. Reading this section was the tipping point — I went to the gym, worked out hard and felt much better. I even tried several new exercises after watching two younger guys doing them.

RETRAIN YOUR BRAIN

The *Wall Street Journal* published an article, "How to Keep a Resolution" by Sue Shellenbarger. Shellenbarger said, "Willpower springs from a part of the brain, the prefrontal cortex, which is easily overloaded and exhausted. What works far better, researchers say, is training other parts of the brain responsible for linking positive emotions to new habits and conditioning yourself for new behaviors."

The main role of the **prefrontal cortex** is its responsibility for **executive function**. We'll get to that in the chapter on exercise and the brain, but let's define it now — the ability of the brain to plan, think clearly and abstractly, and lead us to behave appropriately in a situation. This certainly includes a new activity such as exercise.

One of the more interesting concepts in the article was that people who make progress in developing new habits or self-control in one area tend to improve in others. Students at the State University of New York in Albany who worked on proper posture or recording food they'd eaten got better at several other tasks on which they were tested. When we take charge of our life it benefits us in ways we hadn't thought of. One lady kept a food journal plus had a personal trainer who read it and kept her accountable for her eating and for exercising. She dropped thirty-seven pounds in four months.

DECIDING

Several decades ago a friend had this message on a plaque in his office: "To Not Decide Is to Decide."

If we do nothing, whatever the issue, we've made a decision. If we take no action to improve our fitness and health, that's a decision. We're saying, "I know that I need to implement a real exercise program if I expect to continue to lead an active life for many years, but I've decided not to do it."

I mention this because I suspect many of us say something like the following to ourselves: "I know that I need to implement a real exercise program if I expect to continue to lead an active life for many years, but I just haven't yet decided when I'm going to do it." Sorry, but you have decided, at least for now. You can always change your mind.

DO YOUR BEST

A friend recommended that I read a book by John Wooden, *They Call Me Coach*; it's the story of his life. Wooden died in 2010, at ninety-nine years old. When he was in his mid-eighties he spoke at a ceremony my friend attended. Wooden talked for over an hour with no notes and quoted poems up to thirty lines long. His audience was enthralled.

He was the first member of the Basketball Hall of Fame to be inducted as both a player and coach. Only two others have since been so honored, Bill Sharman and Lenny Wilkens. His ten NCAA National Championships at UCLA in a twelve-year period are unmatched by any other college basketball coach.

There are whole books of his quotations. One of my favorites is, "Success is the peace of mind which is a direct result of self-satisfaction in knowing you made the *effort* to become the best you are capable of becoming." Wooden said — and meant it — that he would rather one of his teams do their best and lose than not do their best and win. How many coaches would say that, much less really mean it?

Our job is to do our best. In fitness, that means we show up, no matter what.

We try new exercises, even if we aren't comfortable — yet — with them. We understand that we'll be sore when we call on muscles that have been dormant. We get over it.

When Wooden died Kareem Abdul-Jabbar, one of his greatest players, said: "Coach Wooden enjoyed winning, but he did not put winning above everything. He was more concerned that we became successful as human beings, that we earned our degrees and that we learned to make the right choices as adults and as parents."

"In essence," Abdul-Jabbar concluded, "he was preparing us for life."

LET'S REVIEW

- Intrinsic behaviors are easy; extrinsic behaviors can be hard. If we stick with extrinsic behaviors, adding frequency and time, they may become intrinsic. Even if they don't they can become a habit.

- Action triggers can be very helpful in both getting going and keeping going.

- Habits are simply behavioral autopilot. We'll develop them if we're patient and persistent.

- Writing down your goals is an important step in achieving them. Sharing them with your spouse and/or friends makes them a commitment. Once you're into it, set a BHAG.

- Written goals are best as short, precise sentences with metrics that are easy to measure. Be sure they have a target date and that your goals are complementary, not conflicting, and focus on a maximum of five goals or less.

- We're motivated by a lot of influences that bear upon us, but we have to make the decision within us to take action. William Ernest Henley said in his great poem, "Invictus," "I am the master of my fate; I am the captain of my soul."

- Help in developing motivation for taking action can come from many sources: our spouse, our views of how others are flourishing, envy of another's good health, maybe even reading this book.

- Kareem Abdul-Jabbar said that Coach Wooden prepared his players for life. That's what we're talking about — preparing ourselves to live a long, healthy, active life.

CHAPTER FOUR — EXERCISE AND THE BRAIN

"You can't change where you came from.
You can change where you are going."—Anonymous

HERE'S WHAT'S COMING

- What's new about the impact of exercise on the brain?
- What's neurogenesis, and what does it mean for you?
- Does exercise impact Alzheimer's and Parkinson's?
- Why should your grandkids start doing aerobic exercise at a young age?
- Does aerobic exercise help stress and depression?
- Does strength training have any effect on the brain?
- What else is important for keeping your brain active and healthy?

If you'd like to retain and even extend your brain capabilities for the rest of your life, please raise your hand. *OK, you can put your hand down now and read this chapter. It may well be the most important chapter in this book — it can change your life.*

One of the more active and exciting areas of research in neuroscience deals with the impact exercise has on the brain. Most of this research is very recent and the end result is mind rattling: aerobic exercise increases cognition. Unfortunately, not enough people seem to be aware of this.

Reading articles and books on the topic has made me realize that it's truly the elephant in the room: not just important but extremely important. When you understand the impact and implications of exercise on your cognitive functions, it hopefully will spur you to take action. It's such a compelling argument to get going.

VERACITY

We've all received messages on the internet that seemed plausible only to learn later that they're completely false. We've developed a healthy skepticism of what we hear and read.

The objective in this chapter is to provide enough information that you'll say, "OK, Harry, I get it; I'm signing up." But I don't expect you to believe me just because I write something on a piece of paper.

There are more quotes and references to scientific articles in this chapter than in any other in order to provide the necessary credibility. This chapter has benefitted from a review by Dr. Art Kramer, Director of the Beckman Institute at the University of Illinois, one of the most important centers for research on the topic of exercise and the brain. I've indicated where he made additional comments to amplify certain sections.

If you encounter an unfamiliar word, check the list of definitions at the end of the chapter. I placed them back there so your eyes won't glaze over, but you do have access to them when needed. We'll discuss some basic concepts of healthy brain function and show how exercise can make your brain healthier — how the care and feeding of your brain can make a difference in the quality of your life.

NEUROGENESIS

Neurogenesis is the process of growth of neurons, or nerve cells, in the brain. For decades the conventional wisdom was that we live most of our lives with the brain cells that we had by the age of say thirty or so. That's no longer the case. *Research has shown that neurogenesis can take place throughout our lives*, although the production of new neurons is reduced as we age. What's the magic potion you take to make this happen? It's not a pill, just our old friend, aerobic exercise.

Hippocampus — that's the section of the brain required for the formation of long-term memory and cognitive maps for spatial navigation. **Spatial navigation** is the processing of information from past and present and using it to make complex decisions. The hippocampus is one of the first regions of the brain affected in the early stages of Alzheimer's disease. What generates neurogenesis in that section of your brain? Aerobic exercise, of course.

One of the products of aerobic exercise is an increase in our ability to utilize oxygen during exercise. The term used to measure our ability to use oxygen is called **VO$_2$ max.** This is liters of oxygen used per kilogram of body weight during intense exercise. Several studies have shown that those with the highest VO$_2$ max also scored the highest on memory testing. The research is clear: Aerobic exercise promotes neurogenesis and lowers the risk of dementia.

Art Kramer added:

"There are some interesting studies with what are referred to as knock out or transgene mice. The mice used in these studies produce massive amounts of **beta amyloid**, a protein associated with the plaques common to Alzheimer's disease. When these animals have access to a running wheel there is a substantial reduction in the production of beta amyloid.

"Carl Cotman from the University of California, Irvine, who is cited later in this chapter, has conducted at least one of these studies."

NEUROPLASTICITY

Neuroplasticity is the ability of our brains to act and react in ever-changing ways. When you learn a new word your brain creates connections, called synapses, to record that word. If you use it repeatedly your brain will increase the strength of the synapses and make a stronger connection. This process is called **synaptic plasticity.**

A **synapse** is a junction that permits a neuron to pass an electrical or chemical signal to another cell. The cells are not physically connected; the signal is passed from one cell to another via electrically charged ions and molecules.

Healthy brains have lots of synaptic plasticity because their "owners" are constantly doing things that stretch their brains — exercise, reading, social engagement and learning new ideas. Synaptic connections are also essential to building long-term memories of faces and words, for example.

Golf coaches remind students that a new swing change will take lots of practice before it becomes established as part of the student's normal swing. That's because the brain needs to build stronger synapses so that the new swing becomes consistent. Golf coach Martin Hall says, "Practice makes permanent." It takes lots of repetitions to make it permanent.

What happens if you learn a new word and then never use it again? Your brain senses that the connection is not being used and prunes it; hence that well-known saying, "Use it or lose it." The same is true for an activity you did years ago repeatedly and then stopped doing; over time you'll lose it. The same will be true for the golf swing change if you don't practice.

If you want to retain something new that you've learned, repetition is the key. If you want to retain some information or skill you currently have, the same rule of repetition applies — do it again and again.

BDNF

BDNF is brain-derived neurotrophic factor. In *Spark: The Revolutionary New Science of Exercise and the Brain* by John Ratey, he calls it Miracle-Gro in the brain. It's the material that makes the synapses grow and prosper due to brain activity.

Exercise elevates the production of BDNF throughout the brain. One of the early researchers to study this was Dr. Carl Cotman, director of the Institute for Brain Aging and Dementia at the University of California, Irvine. Cotman's work with mice showed increased levels of BDNF in the hippocampus as a direct result of exercise. The farther the mice ran, the higher the levels of BDNF. Remember what we said earlier: the hippocampus is one of the areas of the brain most affected in the early stages of Alzheimer's.

Cotman said, "One of the prominent features of exercise, which is sometimes not appreciated in studies, is an improvement in the rate of learning. It suggests that if you're in good shape you may be able to learn and function more efficiently."

Art Kramer added: "There are actually several of these neurotrophins that have been associated with increased exercise. In addition to BDNF, insulin-like growth factor-1 and vascular endothelial growth factor are increased with exercise."

OF MICE AND MEN — AND WOMEN

Scientists love to work with mice or rats — laboratory rats, not the creepy kind found in alleys. They can take a bunch of the little guys, put one group in a high activity environment with lots of exercise and another group in a sedentary environment where they just eat and sleep.

After a few weeks or months they dissect them and examine what's happened to their brains based on which environment they were in. What they find is that there's more going on with the active guys than those in the sedentary environment — by a lot.

To be sure that what they learn applies to us, all they have to do is find human volunteers who are either willing to do lots of exercise or just sit — finding those is not all that hard. But then, they need to do a bit of brain dissection. Where did those volunteers go?

As mentioned earlier, the Beckman Institute at the University of Illinois is one of the laboratories generating lots of research on exercise and the brain. Bill Greenough's pioneering studies on the effects of exercise and environmental stimulation on rats was done there.

In the following section we'll discuss two areas of the brain: **dentate gyrus,** which is a section of the hippocampus that contributes to new memories, and **olfactory bulb,** the section involved with the perception of odors.

WORTH READING TWICE

Art Kramer, director of the Beckman Institute, said, "Both the animal and human research is pretty solid with respect to the fitness effect on brain structure, brain function, neurochemistry, learning, memory and cognition." This is from a paper, "The Science of the Brain: A Beckman Perspective" by Steve McGaughey, May 2007. Beckman is the source of many of the studies that examine fitness training effects on human brain structure and function.

Stanley J. Colcombe and others at the University of Illinois reported on fifty-nine healthy but sedentary volunteers, age sixty to seventy-nine. For six months half of them did aerobic exercise and the other half did toning and stretching.

Using MRIs they reported: "Significant increases in brain volume in both gray and white matter regions were found as a function of fitness training for the older adults who participated in the aerobic fitness but not for the older adults who participated in the stretching and toning."

After six months of aerobic exercise that group had the brain volume of people three years younger. They reversed brain loss.

Their conclusion: "These results suggest a strong biological basis for the role of aerobic fitness in maintaining and enhancing central nervous system health and cognitive functioning in older adults."

Another study at UCLA of ninety-four people in their seventies showed that obese people have eight percent less brain tissue that those of normal weight. Their brains looked sixteen years older than the brains of lean participants.

Justin Rhodes, also at the University of Illinois, said, "We know that there are areas of the brain that continuously generate new neurons throughout adulthood and one of those areas is the dentate gyrus section of the hippocampus. It turns out that exercise produces a tremendous increase in the number of new neurons that are found in that area."

Research has shown new neurons in the dentate gyrus and in the olfactory bulb. Art Kramer said, "Every other area of the brain is highly debatable, but these two areas are not debatable. And those neurons are born as a function of exercise."

Art Kramer added: "Actually, although neurogenesis occurs in developed organisms in both the dentate gyrus of the hippocampus and the olfactory bulb — thus far only exercise-related neurogenesis has been found in the hippocampus."

EVEN COUCH POTATOES CAN BENEFIT

A study conducted at the University of Illinois by Art Kramer, Edward McAuley and Michelle Voss followed sixty-five adults aged fifty-nine to eighty who joined a walking group or a stretching and toning group for a year. The walkers moved at an aerobic pace, approximately seventy percent of their MHR (maximum heart rate).

At year's end the walkers had significant improvement in **DMN** (default mode network). DMN dominates activity when a person is least engaged with the outside world — just observing or daydreaming or thinking — that's using their brain during passive activity times. Better DMN means better performance at tasks like planning, prioritizing and multi-tasking.

They also had increased connectivity in parts of the brain related to performing complex tasks and did better on cognitive tests. The stretching and toning group did not do nearly as well.

All of the evidence points to aerobic exercise providing the keys to the brain kingdom. This study seems to show that even while a little is good, more is better. To retain the benefits, you have to keep it up. This is not a case of "I've done that, now I can go back to my old habits."

WALKING AND YOUR BRAIN

Kirk I. Erickson at the University of Illinois did a study of 299 dementia-free people who recorded the number of blocks they walked weekly. Brain scans were taken nine years later and after four more years they were tested to see if they had developed cognitive impairment or dementia. Erickson began the work while at Illinois as a post-doctoral student and completed it as an assistant professor at the University of Pittsburgh. They found that those who walked seventy-two blocks per week, equivalent to six to nine miles, had greater brain volume that those who walked less.

Erickson said, "Brain size shrinks in late adulthood, which can cause memory problems. These results should encourage well-designed trials of physical exercise in older adults as a promising approach for preventing dementia and Alzheimer's disease." The study was published in the journal *Neurology*.

JACK'S MEMORY

Jack is a neighbor in Bucks County, PA; now in his early eighties, he played on the tennis team at Cornell in the late 1940s. Then he graduated, started working, married and had kids. He did little exercise other than occasional recreational tennis and golf.

Two years ago Jack noticed he was having memory problems. He likes to work *The New York Times* Crossword Puzzle. For those who aren't familiar, it gets harder each day of the week. Historically, Jack was able to complete Monday, Tuesday and most of Wednesday. Over time, however, he found he was having trouble completing Tuesday, much less Wednesday.

Jack went to his gerontologist, who practices at a major university hospital. The gerontologist tested Jack and informed him that he had mild cognitive impairment. He suggested that Jack might want to exercise. Jack says this recommendation was very casual. Note this is from a gerontologist at a major teaching hospital.

Jack decided to do some research. He went home, accessed Google and obtained information that suggested aerobic exercise would be very helpful to him. He went to a nearby gym, signed up and started walking on a treadmill. He kept it up for three days per week without fail. *In a short time he found his memory was improving; he could work Monday, Tuesday and most of Wednesday's crossword puzzles again.*

Then, cold weather set in, dark days, and Jack missed a week at the gym and then another. You know the rest; he gave up. In a short time he was having problems with the crossword puzzles again. Also, some syntax problems got worse. He couldn't get his words in the right order in a sentence.

After a few months' hiatus, he got back with the program — three days a week, no excuses. Soon he and the crossword puzzles became friends again.

Now he's having some coordination and muscle control problems and asked me if I thought strength training would help. I said, "Absolutely." I suggested he hire a trainer so that he learns the best exercises and techniques in order to maximize the benefits.

Scientists likely would not accept Jack's results as fact as there were not enough participants nor was his exercising for a long enough time. But I don't think that matters to Jack; he's a believer.

Art Kramer added: "There is some recent evidence which suggests that resistance (strength) training might also positively influence different aspects of cognition."

BMP + EXERCISE + NOGGIN = NEUROGENESIS

Two terms you need to know for this section: **BMP** (Bone-Morphogenetic Proteins) can be bad guys — a high level of BMP is a major factor in cancer; and **Noggin**, a brain protein that fights BMP. The more Noggin you have, the better. We discussed neurogenesis earlier — the growth of new brain cells. BMPs can also be good guys, necessary for the formation of bone and cartilage, but too much or even too little seems to cause problems.

Gretchen Reynolds of *The New York Times* published an article on July 7, 2010:

"In the late 1990s, Dr. Fred Gage and colleagues at the Laboratory of Genetics at the Salk Institute in San Diego elegantly proved that human and animal brains are able to produce new brain cells and showed that exercise increases neurogenesis."

In a more recent study Dr. Jack Kessler, chairman of neurology at Northwestern University, and others on his staff found that exercise has a major impact on BMP, reducing its effect on the brain. BMP has a negative impact on the growth of stem cells, the precursors for new brain cells. We need stem cells. The more active BMP is in our brain, the slower and less responsive we become as we age.

The good news is that exercise counters some of the effects of BMP. Dr. Kessler and his staff found that mice that exercised on running wheels had fifty percent less BMP within a week. The other good news is that the active mice were found to have an increase in Noggin, the BMP antagonist that improves the amount of stem cell division and neurogenesis.

Dr. Kessler said, "*If ever exercise enthusiasts wanted a rationale for what they're doing, this should be it. Exercise, through a complex interplay with Noggin and BMP, helps to ensure that neuronal stem cells stay lively and new brain cells are born.*"

GOOGLE AND PARKINSON'S

Only one percent of us will contract Parkinson's disease, but if we're one of the people in that group it's a huge issue. Most of us know the story of Michael J. Fox developing it at age thirty. Here's a story of another well-known man who's taking action to increase his chances of dodging this bullet.

Sergey Brin's company Google set a record — the company went from no revenue to twenty billion — in eight years. *Wired Magazine* wrote a lengthy article about Brin, one of the two founders, in their July 2010 issue.

His wife, Anne Wojcicki, founded a genetics company in 2006, providing him with the opportunity for an early look at his genome. He learned that he has a gene called LRRK2 buried within each cell in his body. It's a genetic mutation associated with higher rates of Parkinson's disease.

Not everyone with Parkinson's has it, nor will everyone who has it get the disease, but the odds that someone with this gene will contract Parkinson's sometime during their life goes up between thirty percent and seventy-five percent compared with the average American, who has a one percent risk. Sergey figures his odds are about fifty percent. His chances are also likely increased by the fact that his mother and an aunt have Parkinson's.

What would you do if you were in his shoes? His net worth is about fifteen billion dollars and he's contributing fifty million to Parkinson's research. "Enough," as he said in the article, "to really move the needle."

What else is he doing? One of the few items associated with lower rates of the disease is exercise. It's not surprising that he's implemented a serious exercise program. Brin estimates that with the combination of exercise, green tea (another link to reduced incidence), diet plus steady progress in neuroscience, he can get his odds down to maybe thirteen percent.

He's also bringing an enormous amount of computer firepower to the problem, changing the way medical scientific research is done. If you want to know more about that, read the article; it's fascinating. Sergey Brin is covering his bets on Parkinson's by doing a variety of things, including a regular exercise program. Shouldn't you?

ALZHEIMER'S

Most of us have a friend, relative or acquaintance with Alzheimer's disease. Some of us know of multiple cases. If one or more are close relatives, we begin to wonder what will happen to us. The likelihood of dementia doubles every five years after age sixty-five. Five million people have Alzheimer's today. But there's really nothing we can do about it, right? It's the luck of the genes.

The good news is that there is something we can do. Remember the hippocampus, that section of the brain mentioned earlier, associated with learning and memory? People who exercise have larger hippocampuses; people with Alzheimer's have smaller ones. While it's unclear that exercise can prevent the disease, it's highly likely that aerobic exercise can delay its onset and its progression. How much exercise it takes is the question scientists are seeking to answer now. To be on the safe side, why not do more rather than less?

Sandra Aamodt, a freelance writer, and Sam Wang of the Wang Lab, Princeton University, reported in an article published by *The New York Times* on November 8, 2007: "One form of training, however, has been shown to maintain and improve brain health — physical exercise. Exercise is also strongly associated with a reduced risk of dementia later in life. People who exercise regularly in middle age are one-third as likely to get Alzheimer's disease in their seventies as those who did not exercise. Even people who begin exercising in their sixties have their risk reduced by half."

Executive function is the ability to think clearly, focus, behave appropriately to the situation and remember details. They reported: "Fitness training slows the age-related shrinkage of the **frontal cortex**, which is important for executive function. There's evidence that most behavioral traits, motor skills, and problem-solving tactics are based in this area of the brain. Exercise may also help the brain by improving cardiovascular health, preventing heart attacks and strokes that can cause brain damage. Exercise causes the release of growth factors, proteins that increase the number of connections between neurons and the birth of neurons in the hippocampus, a brain region for memory."

A book covering this topic is *The Roadmap to 100: The Breakthrough Science of Living a Long and Healthy Life* by Walter Bortz. He quotes Dr. Ronald Petersen, director of the Alzheimer's Research Center at the Mayo Clinic: "Regular exercise is probably the best means we have of preventing Alzheimer's disease today, better than medications, better than intellectual activity, better than supplements and diet."

Joe Rojas-Burke reported in *The Oregonian* on January 11, 2010, about a study done at the University of Washington School of Medicine. They had thirty-three men and women who had been diagnosed with mild cognitive impairment, which often leads to Alzheimer's.

Twenty-three of the volunteers began an intense aerobic exercise program, forty-five to sixty minutes four times a week. The other ten spent the same time doing stretching and balance exercises but no aerobics. After six months the aerobic exercisers had significant gains in mental agility while the non-aerobic group had continuing decline in the same tasks. Note that these results are similar to those recorded by Stanley J. Colcombe at the University of Illinois mentioned earlier.

> Fitness clearly plays a key role in lessening cognitive loss. Art Kramer said, "What the research suggests, not uniformly but very consistently, is that if you're fit at time one with everything else being equal — equal education, socioeconomic status, many other factors — that you will have better cognition, better memory, better decision making at time two, and the probability of your being diagnosed with Alzheimer's or vascular dementia will be diminished."

THE SCIENTIST

I met Ted in 1974, at the University of Illinois. He was writing a general chemistry textbook and I was a manager for a publishing company that was interested in acquiring his book. We were fortunate to be chosen by Ted to be the publisher of his book. Since 1977, it's been the best seller in the field almost every year. It's one of the most successful college textbooks ever published.

In 1974, Ted was slim, trim and athletic — he played squash and was a runner — and today he's still slim, trim and athletic. He gave up squash some years ago, has since focused on running and general fitness. He weighs the same as he did in 1974. Today, in his early eighties, Ted still competes in races, generally 5K or 10K. And he does well, but how much competition does he have? He said:

"But you see, that's just the point! I should have more — I perhaps should be competing with you or someone you know who's about eighty. I'm a little lonely in my age group because too many men my age have given up being active, given up keeping fit. Running in races is not for everyone, of course, but there are a lot of good choices for older men to help them stay fit."

Ted and his original co-author have added co-authors in recent years but Ted still plays an active role. He recently told me that he, the senior author in age and longevity, was the one urging the most innovation in the next edition.

Is there any correlation between Ted's exercise regimen and athleticism and his ability to continue, in his eighties, to play such an active role in writing a science book in a highly competitive market? What do you think?

AEROBICS IS THE KEY

The evidence is strong that the most important exercise we can do to stimulate our brains is aerobics. Gretchen Reynolds of *The New York Times* reported September 16, 2009, on several studies that substantiate this view.

She quoted an article from the *American College of Sports Medicine* in which twenty-one students at the University of Illinois memorized a string of letters and then picked them out from a list. After that, they were instructed to sit, lift weights or run on a treadmill for thirty minutes. They then cooled down for thirty minutes and retook the test. They came back for several more days and rotated their activities. In each case those who did aerobics performed better. The author of the study, Charles Hillman, said, "There seems to be something different about aerobic exercise."

One investigator in the field, Henriette van Praag at the National Institute on Aging, said, "It appears that various growth factors must be carried from the periphery of the body into the brain to start a molecular cascade there." Aerobics does it.

BEST IDEAS

A friend, also named Art, said: "One of the things we did almost every day at Mavic (a bicycle component manufacturer) when we were in West Chester, PA, was to have a group lunchtime bike ride. We had twenty-one employees, thirteen of them in key positions. We rode almost every day. During those years we were the leading company in our category. I think that exercise played a part in the ability of those employees to function at a higher level than many of our competitors. Many of our best ideas came during discussions on the lunchtime ride."

FOR YOUR GRANDKIDS

A recent book is *Spark: The Revolutionary New Science of Exercise and the Brain* by Ratey and Hagerman, published in 2008. Early in the book they tell the story of a revolution in fitness at the Naperville School District in Naperville, IL.

Almost twenty years ago the Naperville School District modified their physical education programs so that they provide an emphasis on cardiovascular exercise versus individual sports. They have elementary and high school students running a mile regularly. The students use a heart rate monitor to be sure they are working at eighty percent to ninety percent of their MHR (Maximum Heart Rate). Their grade is determined by how hard they're working, not by a comparison of their performance to any other student. The emphasis is on fitness versus sports.

The results have been dramatic for both physical fitness and academic performance. Some examples:

- Elementary school kids who participated in the fitness program showed a seventeen percent improvement in reading and comprehension versus less than eleven percent for those who did not.

- In 1999 on TIMSS, an international test administered every four years, Naperville High School students finished first — in the world — in science, and sixth in mathematics.

- Thirty percent of U.S. schoolchildren are overweight and another thirty percent are close to it. In 2001, ninety-seven percent of the students in the Naperville district were at a healthy weight as measured by body mass index guidelines.

- In 2005, a team performed a random test of 270 Naperville students, from sixth grade through high school. Only one male student out of 130 was obese. Ninety-eight percent of the students passed the fitness variables.

Naperville has a high socioeconomic demographic with lots of technology companies in and around it. These results, however, signal effects too extensive to be accounted for by socioeconomic factors alone.

The California Department of Education has done studies showing that students with higher fitness scores also have higher test scores.

Why is physical education one of the first subjects to be eliminated when there is a budget crisis? Physical Education departments ought to be flooding their school boards with this information.

Back to the title of this section, "For Your Grandkids"; fewer elementary and high schools today require physical education, much less have an active fitness program. Be sure your grandkids are actively involved in fitness activities, not just sitting on a bench waiting their turn to hit a baseball. Give them a heart rate monitor versus a computer game.

Serve as a role model for them by your own behavior, yet another reason to get going. Ben Franklin said, "A good example is the best sermon."

MORE FOR YOUR GRANDKIDS

Young kids who are fit tend to have bigger brains and perform better on memory tests than their less-fit peers. Think about that one for a minute, Grandma and Grandpa.

Art Kramer, Laura Chaddock and Charles Hillman, all of the University of Illinois, did a study involving forty-nine nine-year-old and ten-year-old subjects to measure the size of specific structures in their brains. The researchers measured how efficiently the subjects used oxygen while running on a treadmill. Chaddock said, "This is the gold standard measure of fitness." Kramer added, "The physically fit children were much more efficient than the less-fit children at utilizing oxygen."

They also used MRIs to measure the relative size of the hippocampus section of their brains and found that the fit childrens' hippocampuses were twelve percent larger relative to total brain size. The more-fit children also performed better on memory tests. They were better able to remember and integrate information than their less-fit peers.

The sooner you can get your children and their children to understand the importance of fitness to their physical and mental health, the better.

USE IT OR LOSE IT

Jay, one of my cycling buddies in Bucks County, is an athletic man in his late sixties. He took up cycling with a vengeance at age fifty and soon was competing in state and national races. He gave up racing five years ago in order to spend more time with his grandkids. He said, "I think they would rather remember me for the time we spent together than for the trophies I won."

Prior to cycling Jay was for thirty-five years a serious tennis player, with a capital "S". He had a national ranking and played against guys like John Newcomb, Jimmy Connors and Bjorn Borg.

Last year, after an eighteen-year hiatus, Jay decided to play a little tennis again. He'd not played for eighteen years. He got out his old racket, had it re-strung and went out to play. He was awful.

What happened? His motor skills, finely tuned for all those years, had not been used. His brain said, "You aren't using these skills anymore so I am going to delete them from your hard drive." Away they went, not to return, unless he's willing to expend a good deal of energy to get them back.

Jay decided to try something new; he bought a baby grand piano and with his wife signed up for piano lessons. Jay had never played a musical instrument in his life. As he said, "Getting the brain to connect what it sees on paper to what the hands need to do is really hard at sixty-eight years old."

Jay is using his brain and will be aided in developing piano skills by his high level of aerobic activity — he cycles over 6,500 miles a year. We were cycling recently and he said, "Off my bike I'm a little old man; *on my bike I'm somebody*." He's justifiably proud of his cycling skills.

EXERCISE AND ANXIETY

I'll assume that you've bought into the concept that exercise generates neurogenesis — the growth of new brain cells in the brain. Another recently discovered concept is that the newly created brain cells may differ somewhat from other brain cells.

Gretchen Reynolds wrote about this in an article, "Why Exercise Makes You Less Anxious," published in *The New York Times* on November 18, 2009. She reported on research done at Princeton University and the University of Colorado.

As usual with such experiments, the Princeton researchers had a group of active rats and another group that had just sat around. They then put both groups in a stressful environment swimming in cold water, not one of their favorite activities. When the researchers dissected them they found that the new brain cells created in the rats that had exercised had somehow been buffered from the stress of the cold water swim.

Then researchers at the University of Colorado found that serotonin, considered a "happy" brain chemical, may not be so happy after all. They did the usual two sets of rats and found that those who had not worked out and were stressed had an increase in serotonin activity while the rats who'd exercised for several weeks had less serotonin but were less anxious in the stressful situation.

Michael Hopkins, a graduate student affiliated with the Neurobiology of Learning and Memory Laboratory of Dartmouth, said, "It looks more and more like the positive stress of exercise prepares cells and structures and pathways within the brain so that they're more equipped to handle stress in other forms. It's pretty amazing, really, that you can get this translation from the realm of purely physical stresses to the realm of psychological stressors."

Now to the big question: How much exercise does it take to generate this wonderful result? The answer is that no one knows. The best course of action, then, is to develop a serious exercise program as described in this book and stick with it for the duration. Clearly one of the most important keys to a healthy brain is aerobic exercise.

GEORGE AND HIS ANTI-STRESS MEDICINE

Here's an example of exercise helping anxiety and stress. George is a real success story. He struggled in high school; he had some learning disabilities but he persevered and graduated. A few years later he started his own business and built it up to the point of operating three shifts, twenty-four hours a day. Then a fire almost destroyed his main factory and he wasn't sure the business was going to survive.

George was feeling lousy and was under great stress. He had headaches daily, stomach problems and was struggling to concentrate and deal with the myriad of problems he had to face. He decided that he wasn't going to allow work and stress to ruin his health. He started running; initially he could hardly run a mile at a slow pace. Within a year he was doing six to eight miles three days a week at a brisk pace and he noticed he was looking forward to doing it.

He found that his headaches went away and also his stomach problems, plus he gained a confidence that helped him deal with the business problems without getting upset. He began looking forward to going to work again. Exercise changed his life and his business.

EXERCISE AND CREATIVITY

A friend gave me the outline of a good story for the book. I liked it but was struggling to come up with a "punch" to it. I decided to think about it when I did a solo bike ride a few days later. I rode for almost three hours and the juices started flowing.

I came up with a title and a theme for the story, wrote it in my head. Then, going up a hill, I recalled an incident when a friend and I cycled up the same hill and had another story; I wrote that one in my head also.

In the last ten miles I happened to think about my favorite uncle who died three decades ago, recalled something that would make a good story. I went home and wrote three stories.

Does exercise help the brain function better? I rest my case.

Roger added: "Harry, these anecdotes remind me of something which happened to me. I've been working on a manuscript on body fat management. Since retiring I've had more time to devote to it. One of the hardest parts was getting the right title. I struggled with several versions, but none ever felt right.

One day on a run I realized that THIN was a central concept and that I might look up all the words starting with "in" and couple them with TH. I now call the manuscript THinsight. I'll be working on this manuscript over the Christmas holidays and would like to send it to you for your feedback."

MILTON AND ROSE

My wife Deb and I love Hawaii and have been there many times. One year we were on the island of Lanai, having dinner in one of the hotel restaurants, when an older couple walked in. They were both just over five feet tall — none other than Milton and Rose Friedman.

Milton, one of the most influential economists of the twentieth century, was awarded the Nobel Prize in Economics in 1976. At the time we saw them they were in their mid-eighties.

I went over to his table, introduced myself and mentioned a couple, Frank and Mary, whom I knew were close friends of theirs as well as mine. Frank and I had worked together for many years and he'd told me about visits with the Friedmans at their summer home in Vermont.

We chatted for a few minutes. I asked about various books of his, some going back decades. His responses were instantaneous and precise. I mentioned a book he'd published with my company three decades ago. He knew the exact title and the year it was published. It reminded me of talking with a very bright thirty year old. The phrase, "A mind like a steel trap" is appropriate.

The next morning I went to the fitness center and noticed two treadmills going, the heads of the occupants barely visible above the control panel. You guessed it; Milton and Rose were there for their morning aerobic exercise. No wonder he maintained his brainpower.

STRENGTH TRAINING AND YOUR BRAIN

The evidence is clear that aerobic exercise has a direct impact on cognition. What about strength training? Some recent evidence suggests that this will help also.

A group of researchers at the Federal University of Sao Paulo in Brazil reported on a study of sixty-two elderly individuals who were randomly assigned to one of three groups for a twenty-four-week period. The control group did warm-ups and stretching plus strength training without overload. The moderate group did the same plus an overload in strength training of fifty percent. The high group did the same plus overload in strength training of eighty percent.

The results were that the moderate and high groups had equally beneficial improvements in cognitive functioning. However, only the high group showed an increase in lean mass in relation to the control group. The impact on muscle strength gain was similar for both the moderate and high groups.

There are limited studies to date similar to this one, but the evidence is encouraging for the role of strength training in retaining and improving cognition.

BRAINS AND BRAWN

Gretchen Reynolds recently wrote an article in *The New York Times* magazine about strength training and brainpower. She reported on researchers in Brazil simulating strength training with lab rats by securing weights to the tails of rats and then having them climb a ladder five times a week. They had another group run on a treadmill and a third group do nothing.

After eight weeks both the running rats and the strength-training rats had much higher levels of BDNF, the ingredient that makes the brain grow and prosper.

Both groups did well on learning and memory. They got smarter.

Some researchers in Japan loaded some running wheels so that the rats had to work harder. The results was that they increased their muscle mass. They also showed increased levels of gene activity and BDNF levels. The harder they worked, the greater the activity.

You may say, "That's very interesting, but I don't happen to be a rat. What's that got to do with me? It's a good question. While there's not a direct correlation of these studies to humans, the speculation is that because strength training strengthens the heart and improves blood flow to the brain there's an improvement in cognition.

Another factor may be that strength training requires more thinking about doing exercises in the correct manner while aerobic exercises tend to be more rote. Greater use of the brain leads to additional brain circuitry.

YOGA AND YOUR BRAIN

A study from Boston University School of Medicine found that doing an hour of yoga three times a week for twelve weeks increased GABA levels by thirteen percent as measured in the study's healthy participants right after a yoga session. GABA, a neurotransmitter in the brain, is lower in people who are depressed.

"This is the first study to find a behavioral intervention — yoga, in this case — that has an effect on brain chemistry similar to that of antidepressants," says study author Chris Streeter, M.D.

ONE THING LEADS TO ANOTHER

Complex activity, like learning to play the piano — or writing a book — has multiple benefits. Not only do you get better over time with the activity but the circuits you've built in your brain can also be recruited for other activity. Someone who learns to play the piano can get better at decision making or solving math problems. I hope the same is true for someone who writes a book.

Ever do something you're not good at? Most of us don't often enough; we tend to avoid such activity. But we shouldn't be so quick to dismiss becoming involved. Not only can we get better at new activities but in the process we challenge our brain to develop more connections.

VARIETY IS THE SPICE

Some of you have likely listened to the popular NPR radio program, "Prairie Home Companion," starring Garrison Keillor. My wife Deb and I went to one of his performances in Philadelphia a few years ago during which he told the story about the farmer and his wife. The farmer's wife said, "That bull of yours has serviced two hundred cows this year; you ought to take note." The farmer replied, "Yeah, but it's not the same cow."

We need variety, too, but in a different way. Exercise, reading, crossword puzzles, Sudoku, movies, social activities — they all contribute to the health of our brains. All of this tells the brain that it's got to keep building new connections.

One study by a Harvard research group identified social engagement as the single strongest factor in the longevity of the group studied, but this doesn't mean that without exercise that they were able to lead an active and healthy life.

A number of companies have developed computer programs designed to challenge the brain and improve its function. If you're interested in exploring this, Google "brain fitness programs." Amazon has a number on their website. Posit Science is a company with a wide range of products in the field. Some city libraries now have them so that you can try them out before purchasing.

In one article Art Kramer at the Beckman Institute expressed the view that they can be good for developing a specific skill, but it's not yet proven that the skill is transferable to other brain functions or to other skills in our lives, such as driving, learning a new language or learning to play a new musical instrument.

A monograph published in 2009, authored by Christopher Hertzog, Art Kramer, Robert Wilson and Ulman Lindenberger said, "We conclude that, on balance, the available evidence favors the hypothesis that maintaining an intellectually engaged and physically active lifestyle promotes successful cognitive aging."

They also said that new studies suggest that some situations requiring executive coordination — complex video games and divided attention tasks — provide training that does transfer to other skills. There's considerable reserve potential in the cognitive skills of older adults that can be enhanced. An intellectually stimulating lifestyle also reduces the risk of Alzheimer's.

Aerobic exercise, intellectual stimulation and strength training — they all have the potential to help us lead an active, healthy life for as long as we're here. I like this quote from a *New York Times* article by Marc E. Agronin, M.D.:

"We will all grow old, and despite the inevitable changes we do have choices.

Indeed, growing evidence suggests that the aging brain retains and even increases the potential for resilience, growth and well-being."

LET'S REVIEW

- The evidence is overwhelming: aerobic exercise has a significant positive impact on brain function. Some recent evidence suggests that strength training also helps.

- Contrary to historical views, today we know that exercise can and does promote neurogenesis as well as aid neuroplasticity.

- The best antidote currently available for Alzheimer's or Parkinson's disease is exercise. No drug treatment comes close. Consistent aerobic exercise has a profound impact on reducing your chances of developing either disease; at minimum, it can delay the onset.

- Staying mentally active, with novel, challenging activities is also useful.

- There's no research yet that's determined the minimum amount of exercise required for impact. Given this fact, more is better.

- Other activities to stimulate your brain are also important — socializing, reading, working crossword puzzles, Sudoku — physical activity and intellectual activity are the keys.

DEFINITIONS:

- **BDNF** (Brain-Derived Neurotrophic Factor) — A protein produced inside nerve cells that fertilizes cells to keep them growing and generates new cells (neurons).

- **BMP** — This is bone-morphogenetic protein, which has been found to contribute to the control of stem cell divisions. The more active BMP is in your brain the more inactive your stem cells, resulting in less neurogenesis. It's necessary and beneficial for its primary purpose, but too much is a problem.

- **Cognition** — The scientific term for the process of thinking.

- **Dentate gyrus** — Part of the hippocampus; it contributes to new memories as well as other functions.

- **Executive function** — The ability of the brain to plan, think clearly and abstractly, and behave appropriately in a situation.

- **Frontal cortex** — This area of the brain is important for executive function. There's evidence that most behavioral traits, motor skills and problem-solving tactics are based in this area of the brain.

- **Glial Cells** — These are very active creatures. They surround neurons and hold them in place, supply nutrients and oxygen to neurons, insulate one neuron from another and remove dead neurons.

- **Hippocampus** — A major component of our brain required for the formation of long-term memory and cognitive maps for spatial navigation.

- **Neurogenesis** — The process of growth of neurons, or nerve cells, in the brain.

- **Neuroplasticity** — The ability of our brains to act and react in ever-changing ways. This is the result of complex processes that occur throughout our life.

- **Noggin** — This is a BMP antagonist that improves the amount of stem cell division and neurogenesis. We want lots of noggin in our brains — and a good brain in our noggin!

- **Olfactory bulb** — The section of the brain that's involved in olfaction — the perception of odors.

- **Synapses** — The junctions between neurons or nerve cells. They connect via electrical activity.

- **Synaptic activity** — The electrical activity in the brain that allows nerve cells to communicate with one another.

- **VO$_2$ max** — The liters of oxygen used per kilogram of body weight during intense exercise.

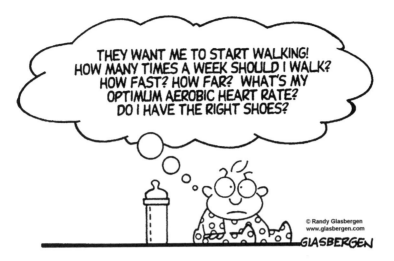

CHAPTER FIVE — AEROBICS: KEYS TO A HEALTHY HEART

"The fitter you become, the better you will be able to live in your body."—Dr. Vijay Vad

HERE'S WHAT'S COMING

- Aerobics: What's the magic about working out in the sixty percent to seventy percent of MHR (Maximum Heart Rate)?
- Krebs — Why should you have any interest in a German biochemist?
- Anaerobics — What is it and why should you care?
- AT — Is it an abbreviation for a state, a medical condition or what?
- Intervals — Why should you do them?
- Heart Rate Monitor — Why do you need one?
- Keeping Records — Why should you write down what you do?

Let's say you're in your sixties, and you play golf three times a week. You view this as exercise — warming up at the range, hitting the little white ball, walking from the cart to the ball and back, raising the glass of beer from the table at the end of the round — all of that burns calories and counts as exercise, right?

Is playing golf better than sitting at home in front of your computer, exchanging emails with your friends? Of course it is. You're burning calories, getting out in nature, socializing with friends, watching the birds. But, it's not enough to impact your fitness level as you grow older. We'll talk about what you need to do to make a difference.

AEROBICS

Just because you're strong doesn't mean you're fit. Dr. Kenneth Cooper, an M.D. in the Air Force, discovered that being strong and being fit are two different things. He found that those who'd done lots of strength training but had not done other fitness exercise did poorly in running, swimming and cycling. He measured sustained performance in terms of a person's ability to use oxygen and coined the word "aerobics," which means "with oxygen."

In 1968, he published *Aerobics*, the first book to provide scientific exercise programs using running, walking, swimming and cycling. It was the first book that provided a scientific basis for aerobic exercise.

Aerobic exercise involves performing an exercise at a moderate level for an extended period. What's "moderate"? That's walking at a pace that gets your heart rate up to sixty percent to seventy percent of your **MHR** (maximum heart rate) and doing it for at least thirty minutes to get real benefit. It's going as fast as you can and still carry on a conversation. You have to consciously work at getting to that level, by the way. We'll cover how to determine your MHR soon.

Here are a few definitions prior to tackling the next section:

- **Glycogen** — It's the main form of our carbohydrate storage, occurring primarily in the liver and muscle tissue. It's readily converted to glucose as needed by the body to satisfy its energy needs.

- **Glucose** — This is the sugar we need for energy. It's transported via our blood and is metabolized by tissues.

- **Lactate or Lactic Acid** — It's an end product of glucose metabolism. It's formed when we are exercising hard and have inadequate oxygen to continue glucose breakdown. We'll use the term lactate.

THE KREBS CYCLE — SIMPLIFIED

There were two big events in 1937; I was born in Albany, Georgia, and Hans Adolph Krebs discovered what's become known as the Krebs cycle. He was awarded a Nobel Prize in 1953 for discovering the biochemical pathways by which energy-rich carbohydrates get converted into the energy we need to keep ourselves going. Nothing newsworthy happened as a result of my being born in 1937, but I still can't help thinking of it as a big event.

When you exercise, the chemical reactions that Krebs discovered kick into gear. Initially energy is generated by breaking down glucose from its storage as glycogen in the muscles and liver. Sustained high-intensity effort will eventually consume all of the glucose.

As glucose reserves diminish, the body relies more and more on fat as its energy source, but it can only do this if work intensity decreases and sufficient oxygen is supplied to allow the working muscles to metabolize the fat. The concept is that glucose and fat are the energy sources, and as intensity increases, glucose becomes the more dominant fuel, though some fat oxidation continues. Since there's a limited amount of glucose available we "hit the wall" when glucose is no longer available as an energy source. At this point we slow down to a metabolic rate at which fat oxidation can be the primary fuel.

At rest the primary fuel is fatty acids. As intensity picks up, glucose contributes a bigger portion of the energy. The intensity of activity determines the mixture of fat and glucose. If glucose is used up, we can continue but only at a slower rate using fat as our energy source.

UNDERSTANDING KREBS

The discussion of the Krebs cycle in this book is highly simplified. Understanding it thoroughly is terrific — if you're earning a degree in biology or chemistry. We don't need to go there.

Let's see if we have the basic understanding that will help us exercise more and better. Following are a series of situations and questions; read and think about them, then review the answers at the end of the section.

We'll use cycling as an example, since that's a sport where it's relatively easy to work in various heart rate zones:

1. We're on our bike, pedaling at a warm-up pace, on the way to meet our friends. Suppose we stay in the fifty percent to sixty percent of MHR range. What's our fuel source or mix — glucose or fat?

2. We meet our friends, take off and accelerate to sixty percent to seventy percent of MHR. Now what's our fuel source?

3. Our cycling group decides to do some intervals; we accelerate from seventy percent to eighty percent, back off to sixty percent, and then accelerate again to eighty percent — we do this four times. What's our fuel source?

4. We're near the end of the ride and all go full speed for a stop sign three hundred yards away. We go all out for as long as we can. What's our fuel source?

THE ANSWERS:

1. The initial source is primarily fat with some glucose.

2. The primary fuel source is still fat, though there's an increasing contribution of glucose.

3. Some fat and as intensity increases shifts to more glucose.

4. We're using the remaining glucose stores in muscles and liver, some lactate is "recycled" and some fat is oxidized. How long we can go depends on our conditioning. When we run out of fuel we "hit the wall" and are done with our speed ride, but we can still make it to the stop sign going at a slower pace using fat as the muscle fuel.

IS THERE A DOCTOR IN THE HOUSE?

If you've been relatively inactive and haven't had a physical exam since your life insurance company required one, get checked out before you ramp up your exercise level. Tell your doctor what you're planning and get his or her approval. If there are some things you should watch out for, better to know before than after.

If you take one of the many beta blockers for high blood pressure or other issues, definitely talk with your doctor before beginning an exercise program. Several of my cycling buddies in Florida take them and exercise hard — with the approval of their doctor. They take the medication after exercising, not before, so that they will have stronger blood flow during a workout. But definitely don't take my word for it, see your doctor.

PREFER LONG OR SHORT?

I'm talking about your life; want to live a long time or a short time? You do have a choice, and what you do determines the outcome. Or you can follow the advice of Charlie Munger, Warren Buffett's partner: "All you need to know is where you're going to die and just never go there." The information below is from a recent newsletter by Gabe Mirkin.

Mitochondria — These are tiny energy-producing chambers in every body cell. They range in number from a few to thousands per cell. It's the enzymes produced by the mitochondria that convert the glucose to energy. They're the good guys; you want lots of them. Unfortunately, they get smaller and fewer as we age. The good news is that exercise stimulates them to produce more enzymes and even to increase and get bigger, both good things.

AMPK — What's this? It's the enzyme AMP-activated protein kinase. This is an enzyme that increases mitochondria in cells. As we age we lose our ability to produce AMPK. That's not good. Exercise increases our ability to make it.

Free radicals — They're the bad guys — we don't want them around for very long. They attach to the DNA in our cells and make them do things that aren't good; think cancer, heart attacks and other bad diseases. Exercise increases the production of free radicals. But there's also good news. Exercise increases antioxidants, which neutralize free radicals.

Antioxidants — They're the good guys; more of them is better. When our body generates free radicals as a result of exercise it also creates **excess** antioxidants to offset them, thereby nullifying them. That's a good thing. The excess antioxidants can help our body offset the effects of free radical exposure from air pollution and smoking, for example.

The message: Exercise is the key to increasing the number and size of mitochondria in your cells, which protects us from free radicals and increases the production of antioxidants.

There are lots of ways you can do aerobic exercise outdoors; brisk walking (nice if some is uphill), cycling, running, cross-country skiing. All should be done at a pace that's near the limit of your ability to carry on a conversation.

Gyms are loaded with aerobic equipment — treadmills (as your fitness improves, it's a good idea to raise the incline at least part of the time), arc trainers, elliptical trainers, stationary bikes, rowing machines. The director of my fitness center in Florida tells me that treadmills get the most usage.

THE TALKERS

I live in SW Florida half of the year and we have lots of walkers in our community. Many, particularly women (they're better at this than men), have a group they walk with regularly. I see the same two women, for example, every time I cycle to meet my buddies for a ride. They're walking at a fast pace, talking and clearly have a good time doing it together.

The important thing is that they're moving at a fast enough pace to get their heart rates up to sixty percent or more.

Aerobics does good things; a stronger heart, improved circulation and lower blood pressure are big ones, really huge benefits. Respiration gets better too. The number of red blood cells goes up, which helps oxygen flow. The chance of getting diabetes goes down, along with the risk of heart disease. Another big plus is how we feel. Aerobics helps build a PMA — positive mental attitude. Serotonin, that feel-good stuff in the brain, gets activated by exercise and provides that sense of well-being.

The more we do, the more our capacity increases and the more it takes to get to that magical sixty percent of MHR. Huh? As we get stronger our system can handle more and our body says, "If you want to work out at sixty percent you're going to have to work a bit harder, because I'm stronger now and I can do more with less energy." The muscle cells get more efficient at using oxygen, which is a big deal; we're getting fit.

BAD NEWS AND GOOD NEWS

Our aerobic power or maximum oxygen consumption — described as **VO$_2$ max** — decreases at the rate of about one percent per year beginning at the age of about twenty. That's the bad news. The good news is that middle-aged men who maintain their activity and body weight show half the decline of their more sedentary friends.

Why did I say men and not men and women? Because a respected study showed that women who regularly exercise had a greater VO_2 max loss than their sedentary women friends. However, the more active still had a higher VO_2 max than the sedentary ones because they started with a much higher number.

WALKING TO YOUR FUTURE

Walking is terrific exercise; it's the only exercise in which participation doesn't decline as we get older. A survey showed that the highest percentage of regular walkers — thirty-nine percent — were men and women sixty-five or older.

Which burns more calories — walking one mile in fifteen minutes or jogging one mile in eight? The answer is that they're about the same. Overweight individuals will burn more calories in either case because they're working harder.

There's walking and there's walking; moving at a slow pace is a stroll. Moving at a pace to get your heart rate going at sixty percent or more is a brisk walk. You'll know it because you'll be breathing deeper and may have trouble carrying on a conversation. Like every other exercise, the more you do it, the stronger you get and the more you can and should do.

Every day there are lots of brisk walkers in our community in SW Florida, but there are some who are out for a stroll. It's better than staying home, but why not pick up the pace a little? Walk at a fast pace for awhile, so that you're breathing hard, then at a slower pace, then back up to a fast pace. That kind of exercise, with structured increases in intensity, is called interval training, and it's really good for you. It gets the blood pumping and the fat burning. Time yourself — begin by doing thirty-second intervals and work up to one minute.

Do you have an iPod? If so, consider going to Prevention.com, then click on Playlists. They have a number of downloads designed for different types of exercise; running, walking, interval training and more. RealAge, another website, is another source. Music can be a good motivator and companion.

Measure the distance you're walking and see how long it takes. A good pace that will get your heart pumping is a mile in seventeen minutes, which is three and a half miles an hour. Set that as a goal if you're not already there, and then shoot for a mile in fifteen minutes.

Bill H suffered a TIA recently — that's often called a warning stroke or mini-stroke — and he's been understandably nervous. He sent an email: "Still being medically tested and all is OK. I'm still walking two and a half miles a day (you started that!) and my wife is joining me!"

THERE'S WALKING AND THERE'S WALKING

Is there any difference between walking at a seventeen- or twenty-minute mile pace on an indoor flat treadmill or outdoors on a flat sidewalk? Think about it for a minute.

If you're on the treadmill you have a motor setting the pace. If you're outdoors, you set the pace with no assistance from a motor. You have to be working harder outdoors than indoors. I don't have a clue just how much harder, but I think it's significant.

Cathy, the director of our fitness center, added: "I agree with your observations... people find it a safer environment — do they just veg out while working out — are they multi-tasking (watching the news, stock market, etc.)? Outdoors you have wind slowing you down and the uneven walkways which can be good since it stimulates the nervous system to make adjustments."

Sometimes the only option you may have is to walk on a treadmill, or it may be your preferred method for aerobic exercise. In order to equalize with the effort outdoors why not speed up the pace to a fifteen-minute mile — that's four miles per hour — and raise the incline of the treadmill a few degrees. That should give you the workout you want and need. This is where a heart rate monitor can tell you a lot about what you are — or aren't — doing.

SPEED MATTERS

A study in the January 2010 issue of the *Journal of the American Medical Association* reported that the speed of walkers was linked to their longevity. This was determined by using information from over 34,000 adults sixty-five years or older. The research was led by Stephanie Studenski at the University of Pittsburgh. Those who walked 2.25 mph or faster consistently had greater longevity than those who walked slower, particularly for those over age seventy-five.

Walking requires a lot of skills and uses many parts of the body — legs, heart, lungs, proprioception and the nervous system. If any part of our body is not functioning properly it can lead to a slower walking speed and may be a leading indicator of trouble ahead. The study showed that those who worked to improve their speed had an increased survival rate. That's one more reason to get out and get moving — at a good pace.

WEIGHT VESTS

Sandy added: "By-the-by, I may not have mentioned weight vests. I tried carrying weights in a backpack to work out harder and a firefighter friend told me about weight vests. They fit comfortably and you can vary the weights from five to over forty pounds. It can mean a lot in a walk, especially if you have a problem with jogging. Your heart rate shows it and it'll make you stronger. After you get used to a set weight then add some more. After awhile you don't really notice you have it on."

I checked online and found you can buy a weight vest for under $30 to well over $100. Some are designed for men and women, others specifically for each sex.

A DETERMINED WALKER

This story is adapted from one in the *Sarasota Herald-Tribune* by Chris Angermann on November 9, 2010:

Frank was and is an avid tennis player. Unfortunately, he suffered his first heart attack during a tennis game in 1992, at the age of forty-two. While he neither smoked nor drank, his father and mother were heavy smokers — his father died of a stroke and heart attack at age sixty-three. Secondhand smoke plus heredity were likely the culprits for Frank's condition.

He continued to play serious tennis and over the next ten years had three more heart attacks, all while playing tennis. He's learned not to push himself so hard but he still plays.

He's become a serious walker — big time. He now lives in Sarasota, FL, where he logs ten to fifteen miles per day at a typical pace of 3.5 miles per hour. Since his last attack in 2001, he's clocked 36,000 miles walking. The results: his last stress test shows that he's grown three new blood vessels in his heart. Frank said, "Walking is the best thing for people in my situation. It doesn't put undue strain on your body."

He's very active both socially and doing volunteer work. I like this quote from Frank: "When you do something to help other people, it makes your life worthwhile."

DO THE MATH

An hour's walk at a brisk pace, three to four miles per hour, will burn about 300 calories. Let's say you sign up for five days per week and make no other change in your exercise or diet. What happens?

If you stick with this you will burn 1,500 calories per week, 78,000 per year; since there are 3,500 calories in a pound that translates into twenty-two pounds. You'll likely miss a few days due to weather, travel, etc., but you do have a choice — you can do more distance on other days to make up for it.

We recently returned from a trip to the Mideast. One of the members of the group was Carlos, a young man in his thirties. He told me that when he finished college he was very heavy because he'd spent too much time eating and drinking. He started walking thirty minutes a day and in a year he dropped fifty pounds. Remember that he was in his twenties with the high metabolism that goes with that age.

HOW MUCH IS ENOUGH?

Maybe you're saying "OK, I get it; I can see where doing more intense exercise will be good for me. But what's the minimum I have to do to get the maximum benefit? The issues are frequency and training volume.

When I pick up a book or magazine discussing fitness I see different numbers; some even say with absolute certainty, "In as little as ten minutes a day." Please don't believe them.

Frequency: How about four days a week of aerobic work? In addition, include some strength training, which we'll get to later. Why not? Got something else that's more important than your health? Remember that we're talking about improving your brain as well as your cardiovascular system and strength.

Training Volume: This is the intensity times the amount of time, or duration. You need to get up to a minimum of sixty percent of your MHR to do real good. Figure that you'll need ten minutes to get up to sixty percent — if you work at it. Hitting this level doesn't happen during a casual stroll — it takes a more determined effort, some huffing and puffing.

Once there, you need to maintain that level for thirty minutes or more. That's the duration.

Information can be motivating for many of us. A pedometer, which you can buy for as little as ten dollars at a discount store, can tell you how much you're moving. We then need to add the measure of energy expended to get into aerobic exercise, our goal. For that you'll need a heart rate monitor, which we'll discuss shortly.

MAXIMIZING HEART PROTECTION

Joe Barnes, Ph.D., is a professor in the Department of Exercise and Sport Sciences at the University of North Carolina, Greensboro. He's an internationally recognized researcher in the field of cardiovascular physiology. He said, "A single bout of appropriate exercise will stimulate the heart to increase the synthesis proteins." He also said, "We have found that exercising at a moderate intensity for sixty minutes provides a considerable improvement in cardio protection." Amounts above that provide modest additional improvements.

Consistency is the key. He added, "When the exercise training stops, the stimulus to increase the synthesis of the protective protein also stops. In less than a week, the level of the protective proteins will return to pre-exercise levels."

Barnes doesn't address the issue of frequency. Is one session of sixty minutes per week at a moderate intensity sufficient, or is it sixty minutes per day? And what is "moderate" versus "intense"? Remember that his focus is only on the increase in the synthesis of stress proteins that provide protection against a variety of physical stresses to the heart.

TO EACH HIS OWN

I asked Roger, a kinesiology professor who teaches the subject at a university in Canada, about how much is enough. Roger said:

"You've discovered one of the fundamental exercise conundrums: how to define exercise intensity and what does it mean. The problem is there are no really clear parameters. What may be moderate intensity for one may be very severe for another.

"It's clear that the more intense the activity, the greater the potential benefit. But the greater intensity requirement for many may end up being too stressful and lead to diminishment of activity down the road; they may decide, 'I don't want to put myself through that discomfort/pain again, so I'm not going to do the exercise.'

"Is it better to do twenty-minute sessions three days a week of high intensity or thirty minutes of moderate intensity five days a week? I lean toward the guidelines of moderation and common sense. Let each person decide which is best.

"The higher intensity might produce a slightly greater benefit, but it may turn an individual off. The moderate will produce benefit, and as fitness improves today's high intensity might become tomorrow's moderation. Plus, the total energy output on the moderate intensity (150 minutes per week versus sixty minutes, plus additional higher metabolism recovery energy expenditure) might also be beneficial in body fat regulation. You could suggest a plan of starting with the moderate intensity protocol and then experiment with a higher intensity bout on occasion.

"Regarding the stress proteins, it would appear that moderate intensity requires sixty minutes to produce significant changes versus thirty minutes for cardiovascular improvement. You could recommend that moderate-intensity exercise be increased to sixty minutes to provide that protection. The individual could stick to the thirty-minute routine but throw in a couple of short, higher intensity bouts (fifteen to thirty seconds) to also produce stress protein benefits.

"There are so many variables: how much time is available? How does higher intensity feel — during the activity, after the activity, the next day? Does it impact on repeating the activity? What is the goal? I like to do everything possible to get people moving and repeating the movement. If this means not so intense, so be it."

ARE YOU FIT?

In a *New York Times* article entitled "On Your Marks, Get Set, Measure Heart Health" by Tara Parker-Pope, published on May 23, 2001, she provided an interesting discussion of how to determine the risk of heart problems. Her article is based on research studies done at the University of Texas Southwest Medical School and the Cooper Institute in Dallas.

A variety of indicators exist to measure the risk of heart disease; blood pressure, cholesterol, triglycerides and obesity are examples. The researchers determined that the level of fitness at midlife is another predictor. They analyzed the fitness levels for over 66,000 individuals using monitored treadmill testing to measure cardiovascular endurance and muscle fatigue.

The data showed that men in their fifties who could run a mile in eight minutes or less and women who could do it in nine minutes or less had a high fitness level. Those who took nine minutes and ten and a half, respectively, were moderately fit. Those slower than ten and twelve fell into low fitness. The difference between high and low fitness risk for heart problems is ten percent for high and thirty percent for low.

The message is that the sooner we take steps to improve our fitness, the better. While walking several times a week at a moderate pace certainly trumps doing nothing, more vigorous activity, like doing intervals at a higher pace during walking, will make a huge difference in future years.

TOO TIRED

Art and Sue live in Sarasota, FL, from November to May. For the past few years they've spent the balance in Acadia National Park in Maine, working at a campground. The weather is nice and cool and they're on Somes Sound spending their free time doing the things they enjoy — kayaking, cycling and hiking. They also meet lots of terrific people.

That's the good news. The bad news is that many days they work pretty hard and at the end of the day they're tired and not excited about exercising. They have a system — one day Art will prod them to do something, the next day Sue. They then go and do one of their three favorites.

Once they get going they feel better and have fun. When they get back they're refreshed, relaxed and ready to have a bit of wine with a nice dinner. They sleep like the proverbial baby.

CYCLING

Cycling is my favorite exercise. I've been doing it for over twenty-five years. As we cycle more we have to expend more energy to get to sixty percent of MHR. Our body gets stronger and it takes more cycling at a faster pace to get to sixty percent and higher. That's a good thing.

It's nice riding with one or more friends because we'll ride faster and farther. We provide each other with motivation and support in addition to socializing. We ride single file in traffic but can frequently ride side by side on the country roads in PA.

Cycling is a wonderful form of a very active kind of exercise. It's not for everyone, but many who try it make it their passion. You need to find a form of exercise that will light a fire under you or within you. Once that happens, it will be easy to stick with it as it becomes fun, not work.

PAT'S COMFORT ZONE

I met Pat in 1987, when she was completing her MBA at Harvard. She was concurrently working part-time for an investment group in New York. She joined the firm full-time that summer and worked with me looking for acquisitions.

Pat is one of those great success stories; a product of Hungarian immigrants, smart — she worked hard in high school and attended Dartmouth. She was at the top of her class there and won the Kemeny Prize her senior year. The prize, named after Dartmouth's former president, John Kemeny, recognizes excellence in writing computer programs.

My favorite immigrant story: Pat's mother, newly arrived from Hungary, met the man at a friend's house who was to become Pat's father. Miklos was recently divorced and twenty years older. Ilona was attracted to him. He said, "I will never marry a younger woman." She smiled and said, "Would you consider making an exception?" And he did.

Pat came for dinner a year ago and we talked about exercise, of which she does a lot. I urged her to get bicycles for herself and her husband and a year later she did. Two weeks later she came down to ride with me on what I call a "training ride."

She said she'd be comfortable with ten to twenty miles. After ten miles

I explained that we now had a choice. We could go one route and do twenty miles or a different route and do thirty. She said she was feeling good and chose thirty.

At mile twenty she was feeling it. We were now at the edge of what she'd done and still had ten more to go and much of that was uphill. Her shoes were too tight and her feet were hurting. We stopped and she took off her socks, which helped. Of course, her legs were getting tired.

At mile twenty-five I asked her if she wanted to take a break. She said, "No, if I stop I may not get going again." We kept going and she made it — tired, thirsty, hot, hurting, but happy. She thanked me multiple times for taking her thirty miles instead of twenty, getting her out of her comfort zone.

WHY DO YOU NEED A HEART RATE MONITOR?

A heart rate monitor allows you to determine what your heart rate is at any given time and a reasonably sophisticated model can tell you how much time you spend at various heart rates, called "zones." We'll get to zones in a minute. You can get one at any sports store for as low as $25, but that model won't tell you how much time you spend in different heart rate zones.

A more advanced model costs about $75. It will tell your current and average heart rate, time spent at various heart rates, calories burned and more. Polar is a popular manufacturer. Their products work fine but their instruction manuals translated from Swedish are a bit obtuse. Their support for product repairs is very good.

The advanced model will allow you to set up your heart rate zones, described below, so that you know how much time you're spending below aerobic — warming up or coasting — and then aerobic and anaerobic. This will tell you whether you're achieving your workout objectives, which is important information.

I'm partial to Garmin products, which are more expensive, because I've used their cycling products for years and have had A+ service and support. Check out their website if you're interested in more sophistication.

Another is Suunto, a company based in Finland. You can find a local dealer or order online at their website or Amazon. Their M-series heart rate monitor sells for about $169 on Amazon. It provides verbal feedback like "exercise day," "next set" or "good workout." This can be motivational feedback for some of us.

Many of us have a GPS system in our cars today. Consider a heart rate monitor as a GPS for your heart. Like a GPS, it tells you where you are right now. It also tells you where you've been and how much work you've done at various levels. As to where you're going, that's up to you.

MHR and RHR — In order to effectively utilize a heart rate monitor you need to either know or estimate your **MHR** (maximum heart rate). We'll discuss how you do this with as much accuracy as possible. We'll also cover how to determine your **RHR** (resting heart rate), which is exactly what it says; your heart rate when you're completely rested.

There's a free newsletter every week authored by Dr. Gabe Mirkin. A recent newsletter covered the alternative ways of arriving at your MHR and recommended the following as the best for men:

MHR = 205.8 – (.685 x Age). Here's an example of a man sixty-five: 205.8 – (.685 x 65) = 161. (*There's a different method recommended for women that's described below.*)

Many of you may have used the old formula for MHR of 220 minus age. In this example that would be 220-65=155, a difference of six **BPM** (beats per minute).

Mirkin reported on a study in 2002, of forty-three different formulae for MHR, which concluded that "no acceptable formula currently exists." The formula above was judged to be the best. The margin of error is due to the fact that it covers a very large population and individual heart rates can vary significantly.

You can determine your RHR by staying in bed when you wake up. Put your heart rate monitor on and look at it after a few minutes. If you don't yet have a heart rate monitor, put your finger on the artery at your throat and count the number of pulses for ten seconds and then multiply by ten. That'll be close enough for openers.

HEART RATE ZONES

What are heart rate zones? They're a measure of the rate your heart is pumping at a point in time in comparison to your MHR. It's a bit more complex than that but not a lot. You need to do some simple mathematics one time only. We're going to use the Karvonen Method to determine heart rate zones as it's been judged the most accurate. Karvonen is a Swedish physiologist whose method incorporates RHR as well as MHR.

The Karvonen Method is: (MHR - RHR) x % + RHR. Here's an example, using a RHR of sixty and MHR of 161 at seventy percent:

$$((161\text{-}60) \times .70)) + 60 = 131$$

You may have arrived at heart rate zones by simply multiplying the percent times MHR. In this example, that would be 161 x 70 = 120, a difference of eleven BPM. Karvonen is more accurate.

Following are zones for a man with a MHR of 161 and RHR of sixty:

Karvonen Heart Rate Zones					
Maximum Heart Rate				161	
Resting Heart Rate				60	
Level	Pct	Pct	HR	HR	Exercise Zones
1	60%	70%	121	131	Aerobic — Beginning
2	71%	80%	132	141	Aerobic — Endurance
3	81%	90%	142	151	Aerobic / Anaerobic
4	91%	100%	152	161	Maximum Effort

FOR WOMEN ONLY

The calculation of the correct exercise zones for women is slightly different. This is a result of a study of 5,500 women conducted at the Northwestern School of Medicine in Chicago. The following formula was found to be most accurate:

206 - (.88 x age) = MHR

For example, the maximum heart rate calculated for a sixty-year-old woman is:

206 - (.88 x 60) = 153

Using the Karvonen method, her formula for seventy percent, assuming a RHR of sixty-two, would be:

$$((153 - 62) \times .70)) + 62 = 126$$

Following are the Karvonen zones for a sixty-year-old woman with a MHR of 153 and a RHR of sixty-two:

Level	Pct	Pct	HR	HR	Exercise Zones
1	60%	70%	117	126	Aerobic — Beginning
2	71%	80%	127	135	Aerobic — Endurance
3	81%	90%	135	144	Aerobic / Anaerobic
4	91%	100%	145	153	Maximum Effort

When you first get into exercise you want to spend a lot of time in the sixty percent to seventy percent of MHR. When you really get into it, you still want to spend most of your time there. As you get stronger, you also want to spend some time at eighty percent and even ninety percent. That's how you get both stronger and faster.

Heart rates, both minimum and maximum, are influenced by fitness level and age with a dose of genetics thrown in for good measure. As we get older our maximum heart rate goes down and our resting heart rate goes up, though both are still influenced by our fitness level.

Pat said: "I got my heart rate monitor and love it. It took me awhile but it is so helpful to know how hard I'm working and I love knowing the calories burned."

HEART RATE MONITORS ON FITNESS EQUIPMENT

Some of you may say, "But the treadmill and other machines I use at my gym have a heart rate monitor built in; all I have to do is put my sweaty hands on the metal plates and I know where my heart rate is."

A fitness director who knows her machines tells me that we should not rely on fitness equipment for accurate heart rate measurement or calorie count. Also, the equipment can't tell you how long you were aerobic and how much time in different zones. So, bite the bullet and spend a few bucks to do it right.

JIM AND MARY

Jim and Mary (not their real names) work out at our fitness center in SW Florida regularly. Jim told me, with considerable pride, that he's there six days per week. The problem is that he could be gaining so much more from the time he's spending there.

Take aerobic exercise; the goal of utilizing a treadmill, arc trainer or whatever your weapon of choice is to get your heart rate up to a minimum sixty percent of your MHR — that's minimum. You also want to spend time in the seventy percent to eighty percent range and even some around ninety percent. Those are the intervals we just talked about; anaerobic training. We'll cover anaerobic training later in this chapter.

The trouble is that Jim wants to read the *Wall Street Journal* while he works out on the arc trainer and reading trumps moving for fitness. Jim moves at a slow pace for whatever period of time it takes him to read the day's paper. He may well spend enough time, but the effort expended doesn't come close to getting his heart rate where it should be.

Mary uses an elliptical trainer. They don't work out side-by-side, so Jim can't see the difference between what he does and what Mary does. If they were running a marathon Jim would be an hour behind. Mary would be on her second beer.

Recently I asked Mary if she wore a heart rate monitor. She said, "Is that the thing you wear on your bicep?" I said, "No, that's a radio. A heart rate monitor strap goes around your chest, measures your heart rate as you exercise, tells you how you're doing. You have a device like a watch on your wrist to give you the information." She said, "Oh." I didn't pique her interest.

That's from a woman who exercises regularly and is in great shape. She can do yoga moves that my body doesn't allow. She does some strength training, albeit with light weights, but if everybody did what Mary does we'd have a much lower national health care bill.

Would Mary benefit from using a heart rate monitor? I think yes. She would know where her heart rate is, could review how much time she spends in each zone and might be motivated to spend more at a higher heart rate periodically.

How about Jim? Are you kidding? He doesn't have a clue where his heart rate is, but I can tell you that it's not where it should be. He's on a stroll and thinks he's running. It's better than sitting at home but not even close to the benefit he could achieve with the same amount of time invested.

You need to know the difference between going through the motions and really doing the work. If you quit just as the burn or breathlessness begins, or when the reps get hard, you're missing the point. The heart rate monitor is almost like having someone look over your shoulder and critiquing your effort. Remember: maximize your time investment.

WHICH BURNS THE MOST FAT?

I've heard more than a few people say that they want to do most of their exercise at a low intensity because that's where they burn the most fat. While it's true that the highest percentage of total energy is derived from fat at low intensity exercise, that's not the whole story.

Say you're out for a walk — more like a stroll — at a leisurely pace that has you working at about fifty percent of your MHR. At that level about sixty percent of energy comes from fat. That's certainly a big percentage.

If on another day you go for a real walk — how about a mile in seventeen minutes, or about three and a half miles an hour — then you're likely working closer to seventy-five percent of your MHR. This will lead to about forty percent of the energy coming from fat. So the stroll trumps the real walk? Not so fast. The reality is that at seventy-five percent of your MHR the energy expended is two and a half times greater and the actual amount of fat consumed is over thirty percent higher.

ANAEROBIC EXERCISE — WHY DO IT?

Anaerobic means "without oxygen," operating at a level where you're breathing hard, going all out. I remember running through LaGuardia Airport years ago, heavy briefcase in hand, trying to catch a flight to Chicago. I made it but couldn't talk when I got to the gate. That's anaerobic. Another would be the feeling after shoveling heavy snow — I lived in Chicago — for ten minutes or more, panting and out of breath. Remember running to the point of being out of breath as a kid? The shorter and higher the intensity, the greater the use of anaerobic energy.

All of our muscle fibers can be divided into two categories: slow-twitch and fast-twitch. We use slow-twitch for endurance, like jogging, walking or cycling long distances at a steady pace. Fast-twitch muscles kick in when we "go anaerobic" or work at a high energy level. Going from a jog to a sprint, or cycling as hard as possible, will do it. Lifting heavy weights is another example of using fast-twitch. We'll talk more about strength training and muscle fibers in the next chapter.

Another big plus to doing anaerobic exercise is that it increases your metabolism and more calories continue to be burned after exercise; your

RMR (resting metabolic rate) may run higher for as long as twenty-four hours. RMR is the amount of energy consumed at rest.

Aerobic exercise uses more calories during the activity because it goes on longer. Your recovery will be faster and enhanced metabolism will be less than during a high-intensity, anaerobic workout. You'll work for a shorter time at a higher intensity, but the longer recovery period means that total energy expenditure and fat use as an energy source will be similar to an aerobic activity.

The increase in RMR can be a real benefit for those who do lots of exercise; they're burning more calories per unit of body weight on a continuous basis than those who aren't fit. Fit individuals have more muscle that's metabolically active, so they have a higher RMR and use more fat energy 24/7 than their sedentary peers.

MORE ABOUT METABOLISM

Gretchen Reynolds wrote an article in *The New York Times* on June 20, 2010, entitled "A Workout for Your Bloodstream." Following are some of the details.

Scientists at Harvard and several other institutions drew blood from a group of fit adults as well as from an unfit group. They also did the same for some runners from the 2006 Boston Marathon immediately after the race. They had the first two groups exercise for ten minutes on a treadmill or stationary bike and then drew blood again.

The fit group had almost a one-hundred percent increase in their metabolites associated with fat burning. The unfit group had a fifty percent increase. The marathon runners immediately after the race had a 1,000% increase. Clearly the more fit the individuals, the more fat they burned.

WHY DO INTERVALS?

A number of you may say, "Harry, I'm not a professional or even an amateur athlete. I'm just an average person who'd like to become more fit by exercising more and eating healthy. Why should I do intervals? That's for athletes."

That's a very understandable point of view. Not too many years ago

I had a similar view about intervals and even about strength training, which we'll get to soon. I didn't see a purpose for intervals and thought strength training would just make me muscle-bound. The good news is that I learned the fallacies in my thinking and made some changes.

Intervals involve doing an activity at a high intensity for a period of time followed by a period of low intensity, then doing it again. The more fit you become, the more you can do. In addition to burning more calories during and after exercise as a result of interval training, you also increase your aerobic capacity, known as VO_2 max — the amount of oxygen you can deliver to your muscles. Individuals with a high VO_2 max live longer, among other benefits. Let's review an example.

Walking — Suppose that you use walking as one of your aerobic exercises and that your schedule is to walk two miles daily at a pace of three miles per hour. This means you're spending about forty minutes per day.

As you improve your fitness level your body will use less energy to cover the same distance. That's the good news; the bad news is that you're not working as hard as you did. In order to obtain the same benefit you need to either walk longer or faster, or both.

If you increased your pace from three to four miles an hour, that should do it for awhile. But, that's a thirty-three percent increase, a big jump. You can "sneak up" on that goal by doing intervals.

After you've warmed up you increase your pace to somewhere between four and five miles per hour for one minute. At the end of the minute you slow back down to your normal pace for two minutes and then accelerate for another minute. Over the course of the two-mile walk you do this five times.

You'll find yourself a bit short of breath during the intervals, which is a good thing. Your heart is pumping faster; you're working harder and burning more fat calories. This process will raise your RMR — resting metabolic rate. This means you'll burn more calories even after you've completed your walk. The higher RMR can last for quite some time, depending on how hard you've worked.

And guess what — by doing this "up and down" walking versus your standard pace all of the time, you'll start walking faster. You may increase your pace from three to four miles per hour in a few weeks of interval training.

Remember that with any exercise, the more we do the stronger we get and the more we need to do to obtain the same benefits. We can accomplish more in the same period of time by doing intervals.

This approach applies to any aerobic activity — running, cycling, rowing, swimming, whatever.

Let's review the benefits: burn more calories, both during and after exercise, increase your oxygen capacity and live a longer, healthier life. Sounds like good reasons to me.

LOTS OF WORK

When we think about how much work our heart has to do for all of our life, it makes sense that we ought to devote some time to its care and feeding. Here's what Bill Bryson said in his wonderful book, *A Short History of Nearly Everything*:

"Your heart must pump seventy-five gallons of blood an hour, 1,800 gallons every day, 675,000 gallons in a year — that's enough to fill four Olympic-sized swimming pools — to keep all of those cells in our body oxygenated. And that's at rest. During exercise the rate can increase as much as six-fold." That, by any definition, is lots of work.

CAR TALK

Ever listen to the NPR radio show, "Car Talk?" Click and Clack, the Tappet brothers, are Tom and Ray Magliozzi, both engineering graduates from MIT. They're smart and very funny.

Recently a woman from California called, complaining that her husband drives by accelerating, then coasting and then accelerating again. Aside from the major discomfort for the passengers, she thinks that the process burns more gas while her husband says it burns less. They agreed to abide by the view of Tom and Ray. At stake was the opportunity for the husband or wife to have bragging rights.

Tom and Ray agreed with the wife that not only did the accelerating, coasting, accelerating process burn more gas, it also generates more wear on the engine. She was delighted.

What the husband was doing is the same thing as intervals. The accelerating, coasting, accelerating process burns more gas or more calories, whether you're dealing with your car or your body. The additional wear on the engine is not good, but it's good when we're giving our body a harder workout. We stress our system and it gets stronger.

RHR MATTERS

Earlier we talked about resting heart rate (RHR). What your RHR is matters, quite a lot. A 2011 article in *The New York Times* by Anahad O'Connor was enlightening on this topic. It reported on a research study involving 50,000 healthy men and women over two decades. The purpose was to determine whether an RHR at the upper end of normal increased the risk of dying due to a heart attack. The normal range is considered to be between sixty and one hundred beats per minute.

It turned out that RHR was a good predictor of a healthy heart. About 4,000 of the study participants died over the twenty years. For each ten beats per minute increase in their RHR the risk of dying from a heart attack increased by eighteen percent for women and ten percent for men. Another study found that those who started with an RHR above eighty were more likely to become obese and develop diabetes over two decades.

What was the recommended action to lower RHR? Aerobic exercise — particularly interval training.

A FORMULA FOR INTERVALS

I hope you agree that you don't need to be an athlete to benefit from doing intervals. Overweight people can benefit significantly — it's the fastest way to stimulate growth of the enzymes that burn fat. You can accomplish this by speeding up for a minute or so several times during a walk. The length and frequency of your intervals can and should increase as you become more fit. Here's the process:

First, build a base. Exercise for three months and spend as much of the time as you can in the sixty percent to seventy percent, or Zone 1 on the Karvonen chart. Pick an aerobics device: treadmill, stationary bike, cycling outdoors, running, etc. Ideally measure, via a heart rate monitor, how much time you're actually in that zone. Many heart rate monitors will allow you to set the zones as described in the Karvonen chart and will record how much time you spend in each zone.

Once you have a solid base of aerobic exercise, move to doing intervals. Accelerate until your heart rate reaches Zone 3 on the Karvonen chart, hold it for a minute and then slow down to your normal pace. Wait a couple of minutes and do it again. Try to do this routine five times during your aerobic workouts that, ideally, will last forty-five minutes to an hour.

After two weeks of doing one-minute intervals, increase the time to two minutes. Try to do five intervals at this pace.

After two weeks of two-minute intervals, do something different; work hard and get to Zone 4 for thirty seconds. Wait one minute and do it again for thirty seconds for a total of six intervals.

In each set of intervals look at your heart rate monitor and see how long it takes for your heart to go down from your highest level to Zone 1. The more you do, the quicker you'll recover. Your heart and cardiovascular system are getting stronger. You'll also find that the pace of your aerobic activity will pick up. You can comfortably move faster at whatever exercise method you're using.

THE MARATHONER

Rusty, one of our regular cyclists in SW Florida, used to run marathons. When I asked him how many he said, "Way too many." One artificial hip and one knee replacement were the result, so he took up cycling instead. When I started doing lots of intervals I chose to explain the process to him one day and he politely told me that he did understand. He did them when he was training for marathons and took over twelve minutes off his total time. I said, "Oh."

KICK IN THE AFTERBURNER

Gina Kolata wrote an article in *The New York Times* on April 18, 2011, "For an Exercise Afterburn, Intensity May Be the Key." It reports on research done by Dr. Amy Knab of Appalachian State University in North Carolina that's worth mentioning for the quality of her research design alone.

Dr. Knab and her colleagues recruited ten men, ages twenty-two to thirty-three, to spend two periods of twenty-four hours each in a metabolic chamber. This chamber measures calories burned by individuals inside the chamber. The men had to be sufficiently fit that they could ride a bike vigorously.

During the first visit the recruits were required to stay perfectly still, sitting in a chair. They moved to eat two meals — served through an airlock — and could do a two-minute stretch in the afternoon every hour. They slept in the chamber from 10:30 PM to 6:30 AM. They averaged 2,400 calories each during their stay.

Two days later they came back — can you believe it — for another session. The same rules applied except that they rode a stationary bike at a high level of intensity for forty-five minutes at 11 AM. They burned an average of 420 calories during the exercise and, over the next fourteen hours, they averaged an additional 190 calories. They increased their total calories burned by thirty-seven percent.

The key appears to be the fact that they worked at a high intensity — at least 70 percent of their VO_2 max — a level where they were unable to carry on a conversation. The intensity and the length were critical. Similar experiments showed that exercising even longer increased the calorie burn afterward, but studies working at only fifty percent of VO_2 max did not produce an afterburn.

Clearly there was an increase in metabolism but the exact reasons why haven't been determined. You don't really need to know in order to appreciate the benefits of working at a higher level of intensity. Once you've built your endurance up to the level where you can work harder, take note.

A "NEW" EXERCISE PROGRAM

Here's a "new" idea for exercise: Get up in the morning, eat what you have left from the night before, put on a loin cloth or whatever and go outside. Start off running at a modest pace for about five miles and then accelerate to running as fast as you can for about a hundred yards. Back off to a modest pace and then accelerate again for about a hundred yards. After five miles or so look for a big rock of about fifty pounds or so, pick it up and carry it back to your starting point. You can then sit down and have a nice meal.

This is what Paleolithic man did on a daily basis millions of years ago in order to survive. They likely burned five times or more of energy compared to today's sedentary lifestyle. The acceleration represents what he had to do to catch a wild animal and the rock was the weight of carrying it back to his camp. I don't think they had an obesity problem.

HEIDI AND INTERVAL TRAINING

I cycle in Bucks County, PA, half the year and the other half in SW Florida. Bucks County is terrific for cycling — country roads, low traffic, rolling hills and still lots of farms. Motorists are used to cyclists and treat us well most of the time.

During the past few years in Bucks County I've seen an attractive blonde woman passing in the opposite direction. She always waves, gives me a big smile, looks like a real athlete and is always going in the opposite direction.

Last summer I noticed a blonde a few hundred yards ahead, thought, "Could it possibly be the blonde beauty?" It was. The only way that I caught up to her was that she was recovering between intervals. I pulled up and she gave me a big smile and said, "Hi, I'm Heidi."

We rode a bit, talked and then she said, "I'm going to do a three-minute interval at anaerobic threshold; want to join me?" What could I say? I started to say, "I'll cover your back," but that might not go over well, so I said, "I'll be on your wheel." I tucked in behind her.

I stuck with her but just barely. She recovered and then said, "Now I'm going to do three minutes at VO_2 max." I said, "Heidi, it's been nice riding with you, hope to see you again soon." I rode on, way behind her, thinking, "Self, if you want to ride with Heidi, you'd best start doing some serious intervals." And I did — lots of them.

A few months later I went back to SW Florida, rode with my buddies there and found I could leave them in the dust at will. As one said, "I don't know what training regimen you're on, but it's working." I ride with the group, periodically take off, do a one-minute interval, slow down and wait for them to catch up. A few minutes later I do another one — six to eight per ride.

We have a new cyclist in our group this year. Rob is in his early sixties and has done five Hawaii Ironmans, including 2009. To say he understands interval training is like saying he can tie his shoes. He's taught me some additional techniques, like getting in the biggest gear while standing up and going hard for a few hundred yards. It hurts, but it hurts *good*, and the more I do it the longer it takes before it hurts.

The only way to get faster is to go faster. And the best way is to go faster for a specific period of time, get to ninety percent and go back down to sixty percent and then do it again. Sooner than you would think your average speed is several miles per hour higher.

THE SWIMMER

Nine years ago Rich was looking for a sport to improve his conditioning and he chose swimming. Here's what he said: "I train in a twenty-five meter pool and when I started I couldn't swim across the pool. But to give you a starting point, stay in the water for thirty minutes and swim as much as you can. You increase the workload and time spent until you reach that magic mile. It doesn't need to be a mile nonstop.

"Within a year I could swim a mile in about an hour. Nine years later, I'm at thirty-two minutes for a mile. Anything under fifty minutes for a mile is, in my opinion, very respectable. Interval training is the best way to increase your swimming speed and improve fitness. Most, if not all, workouts should include interval training."

WHAT'S "AT" ALL ABOUT?

Stick with me, I promise not to get too technical. **Anaerobic Threshold** (AT), sometimes called **Lactate Threshold** (LT), is the point in exercise at which lactate starts to accumulate in the bloodstream and limits performance. That's because we're using greater and greater amounts of glucose as the energy source. Since there is limited storage of glucose we deplete our reserves.

The work intensity is such that we can no longer provide enough oxygen to the working muscle cells to utilize the lactate that's accumulating with increasing glucose use. We've shifted into mostly anaerobic metabolism. We've used all of the glucose available and now start building up lactate. This level of activity moves beyond the fat-burning stage.

Take Rich as an example: When he goes as fast as he can, swimming for a minute or more, getting up to ninety percent or Zone 5, he uses up the available glucose in his fast-twitch muscles, which are the ones activated by this burst of speed, and starts accumulating lactate. That's why intervals hurt for a short time period. He can feel it in his arms and legs.

Then, when he backs off and goes down to sixty percent or Zone 1, he gives his muscles time to recycle the lactate and the pain goes away. He's ready to do another interval in a few minutes.

Like any exercise, the more we do, the stronger we get, the more we can do in the future. That's the beauty of working hard. Our body adapts to the new requirements, signs up for a more advanced program. Isn't it a wonderful device? As fitness increases you can go longer without the burn of lactate and can recover quicker. Another benefit is that you can raise your average speed without discomfort.

About thirty years ago Jane Fonda did a very popular aerobics video — remember videotape? Toward the end when she was working hard she said, "Go for the burn." AT is what she was talking about.

DOING THE LACTATE SHUTTLE

Here's some interesting science that corrects a former widely held view of the role of lactate. *If you'd like to learn about it, read on; if not, you can skip this section.*

The conventional wisdom for many years was that lactate was a waste product and served no useful purpose after it was formed. It was even viewed as an exercise-limiting entity. Now scientists recognize that lactate is a valuable fuel source.

The Lactate Shuttle is the process of formation of lactate in one cell compartment during anaerobic exercise, which is then used in another cell compartment, or by adjacent muscle fibers as an aerobic energy source, or by the liver to reform glucose.

During all forms of exercise, glucose is broken down anaerobically to a substance called "pyruvate." As work intensity increases, the amount of pyruvate formed increases. For the muscles to continue to break down glucose, the pyruvate must be cycled into the Krebs cycle or converted to lactate and removed from the cell.

Some of the pyruvate is converted to lactate, which diffuses out of the muscle cell and is picked up by adjacent muscle cells, or it diffuses into the blood where it can be transported to distant muscle cells or the liver.

If the exercise intensity is low enough the lactate doesn't accumulate within the muscle cell or in the blood and there are no side effects. However, if the exercise intensity is too great the lactate builds up within the muscle cells and blood, changing the pH and interfering with cell metabolism. This creates the "burning" sensation associated with "lactic acid buildup."

In the Lactate Shuttle the lactate formed as glucose is broken down. It can enter into the Krebs cycle in adjacent and distant muscle cells, to be used as an energy source during aerobic oxidation. This spares muscle glycogen use as an energy source. The lactate can also diffuse into the blood and circulate to the liver where it is converted back into glucose. The newly formed glucose can be put back into the circulatory system and taken up by distant muscles to be used as an energy source, or it can be stored in the liver as glycogen.

Lactate is a necessary and important by-product of glucose breakdown during muscle activity. As fitness improves the ability of our body to "shuttle" lactate increases. We're then able to work at a higher intensity without feeling the negative side effects of lactic acid buildup.

LONGER IS BETTER

I'm talking about **telomeres**, of course. A telomere is a short stretch of repetitive DNA at the end of the DNA strands that make up the chromosomes.

Three scientists — Elizabeth Blackburn, Carol Greider and Jack Szostak — won the 2009 Nobel Prize in Physiology or Medicine for the discovery of how chromosomes are protected by telomeres and the enzyme telomerase.

Your logical question about now is, "So what?" I'm glad you asked, and I promise not to get too technical in answering. Gretchen Reynolds had an article in *The New York Times* in 2010, about telomeres, short and long, and how they relate to fitness and life expectancy.

The telomeres at the end of DNA strands shorten each time a cell divides. Eventually there's no telomere left, so the cell either dies or enters into senescence — that's aging. The longer the telomere, the longer its life; the more long telomeres we have, the better off we are.

Remember the phrase, "Youth is wasted on the young"? It fits here. Both active and inactive young people were compared by some German scientists, one of whom was Dr. Christian Werner, an internal medicine resident at Saarland University. Young adults in their twenties have telomeres of about the same length, whether they do lots of exercise or very little.

"But I'm not young anymore; what happens as we get older?" Good question. They found that middle-aged, relatively inactive adults had telomeres forty percent shorter than the young subjects. They also found that middle-aged adults who were very active physically — longtime runners — had telomeres only ten percent shorter than the young guys. So telomere loss was reduced by seventy-five percent in the older athletes. As Dr. Werner said, "Exercise, at the molecular level, has an anti-aging effect."

Thomas LaRocca, a Ph.D. candidate at the University of Colorado, tested people fifty-five to seventy-two years old for their VO2 max — their maximum aerobic capacity — and the length of their cells' telomeres. He found that the higher the VO2 max, the longer the telomeres. Did I mention that your VO2 max is a strong indicator of your fitness? Those who exercise have both higher VO2 max and longer telomeres.

How much exercise is enough to provide significant benefit? That's uncertain, but scientists do know that long-term endurance training is associated with a slower rate of telomere erosion compared with those who do not exercise. As Dr. Werner said, "Any form of intense exercise that is regularly performed over a long period of time will improve telomere biology."

Now keep in mind that the role of telomeres in aging is still quite new. Notice that the Nobel Prize was awarded in 2009. This is still a hot research topic. What we do know up to now, however, provides one more intriguing link between cardiovascular fitness, overall fitness and longevity.

SUB-AEROBIC

You're going to spend a good deal of time in most forms of exercise below your aerobic zone, what I call sub-aerobic. Energy will be expended in the sub-aerobic zone and working at that level is part of the process of fitness development. Why? Here are a couple of examples:

A not-so-fit person starts an exercise program by committing to a forty-five minute walk four days a week; that's about two miles each day. Let's say the first half-mile has a downhill slant. He or she likely will not reach their aerobic level in that distance. If the next half-mile is slightly uphill, they should get there. And if they turn around to come back the same route, the reverse happens. If they're not real fit, half the time will be aerobic.

Those in the fit category spend lots of time in the sub-aerobic zone. A fit solo cyclist will likely be aerobic or anaerobic for less than half of the length of his ride. It takes more effort to get up to that level. His body is accustomed to exercise and it doesn't work very hard until he really cycles hard. He can't "go aerobic" when cycling downhill — it simply won't happen. Once he hits an uphill incline or a real hill, then things start happening. If the road is flat, he has to work hard to become aerobic.

Is the time spent sub-aerobic a waste? Not at all. We're burning calories, getting the blood flowing, moving the body. Factor this into the time spent so that you allocate enough time to achieve your training objectives.

That's why cycling, walking or jogging with one or more friends is so beneficial. There's no question that we work harder with others than we do alone, plus it's more fun to have someone to talk to. Making exercise social as well as physical adds motivation for showing up.

EXERCISE OR MARIJUANA?

Gretchen Reynolds wrote an interesting article in *The New York Times* in 2011, about the role of endorphins in producing that feeling of euphoria that can accompany intense or prolonged exercise. Endorphins have for decades been given credit for that feeling. The problem is that endorphins are relatively large molecules, too large to pass the blood-brain barrier. Having endorphins in the bloodstream after exercise doesn't mean that they were having an impact on our brain.

A 2003 study at the Georgia Institute of Technology showed that fifty minutes of hard running on a treadmill or riding a stationary bike significantly increased the levels of endocannabinoid molecules in a group of college students. The endocannabinoid system was discovered some years ago when scientists were studying how marijuana affects the body. They found that certain receptors allow marijuana to initiate reactions that reduce pain and anxiety plus produce that sense of well-being. They found that the body can create the same results via endocannabinoids. These are small enough molecules that they can pass into the brain.

Further studies with laboratory rats have shown a probable role of endocannabinoids in not only providing that sense of euphoria but also to our enjoyment of exercise. Rats aren't very talented at filling out questionnaires, but the data from them is very interesting. Given a choice of marijuana or exercise, I'd suggest you choose exercise. You can achieve the same result without the worry of being arrested.

SPORTS DRINKS

When we exercise for a long period of time we can deplete our store of carbohydrates in our muscles and experience fatigue. Can drinking sports drinks that include carbohydrates have a positive effect on performance? The answer is a definite yes for longer-duration exercise, those of sixty minutes or more.

We're talking about sports drinks, not the high-caffeine energy drinks available in many stores today. An example is Gatorade, available in a wide variety of stores. Many of the sports drinks are available in powder form at athletic stores, bike shops and even some grocery stores.

Begin drinking fifteen to thirty minutes after exercise is started and drink five ounces every fifteen minutes. It's also good to use another product after an intense workout or bike ride to speed recovery. The sooner you eat or drink carbohydrates after exercise, the more effective your recovery. Some of the products for this purpose are Recoverite, Endurox and Ultragen.

Studies have shown that ingesting protein immediately after a hard workout, along with a carbohydrate drink, can speed the recovery process even more.

WHAT ABOUT MILK?

Researchers have recently provided support for the fact that milk may be as good — or even better — for recovery from an intense workout. How about that; I guess our mothers were right in urging us to drink lots of it many decades ago.

Milk has carbohydrates, electrolytes, calcium and vitamin D, but it also has two ingredients that help us regenerate muscles fast — casein and whey proteins. A nutritionist at the Medical Research Council in the U.K. said, "Milk provides the building blocks for what you need to build new muscles." She said that sports drinks often don't have the nutrients to regenerate muscles. The scientists recommended low-fat milk as best.

There must be something to this; Michael Phelps drank a flavored milk drink at the Beijing Olympics, where he won six gold medals. At the Vancouver Olympics dairy farmers brought in 85,000 quarts of chocolate milk for their athletes. Did it help? Well, the Canadians won a record fourteen gold medals. I haven't tried it but I'm going to after reading this. My friend Art has been using chocolate milk for workout recovery for years and swears by it.

REST AND RECOVERY

Let's say you do a hard aerobic workout on Monday — cycling, running, treadmill, whatever your exercise of choice. At the end you're tired; happy tired, but still tired. So, if you want to be fit and strong, you should do it again the next day, right? No. Our bodies need time to recover from the stress of exercise. Make the next day less intense in terms of effort or time. Even better, make it a day at the gym doing strength training.

Determine a schedule that works for you. Maybe Sunday, Wednesday and Friday are aerobic days. Tuesday and Thursday are for strength training. Monday and Saturday can be for a less strenuous activity like golf or doubles tennis.

Listen to your body. If you're scheduled for an aerobics workout and don't feel good, take it easy. Maybe go for a walk instead of running, cycling or doing aerobics at your gym. The following story is a great example of hard and light days.

CLIMBING MT. WASHINGTON

Neale is a resident of Camden, ME. Mt. Washington in New Hampshire is the highest peak in the northeast. *The highest surface wind ever recorded on earth was on the summit of Mt. Washington; 231 mph on April 12, 1934.* Neale is in his mid-sixties, Ned in his early twenties. The climb was in October 2010.

"This weekend Ned and I put to the test the concept of working to exhaustion. Climbing Mt. Washington in extreme conditions really took it out of both of us. Good thing we turned around when we did (about half a mile from the summit when visibility was down to 100 yards and the wind was a steady fifty knots with gusts, according to the radio, of sixty to seventy — enough to knock us down), because by the time we got back to the parking lot, our legs were jelly.

"The next day Betsy and I did a short two-mile hike up one of the local mountains in Camden, about 800 feet of vertical (vs. 2,800 vertical on Mt. W). That took some of the soreness out. And today I'm going to the YMCA for a light workout.

"When I say we went to exhaustion, I'm not kidding. This was near total exhaustion, but after a light day yesterday and a good square meal of roast beef, veggies and mashed potatoes, I feel great today.

"Walking up the hill across the street today with my dog Tucker, I could feel a spring in my step that I haven't felt for years. It felt as if my heart was working noticeably less hard to walk up the hill. At the top I wasn't even breathing hard, which was not the case last week before the climb. All because I had gone to exhaustion and then had a light day."

While Neale is in his mid-sixties, he's been in a serious exercise program for decades, including lots of hiking in the hills around Camden. This story is a testament to his condition and the power of exercise to allow him to perform at the level described.

WHAT'S YOUR PASSION?

It certainly helps if you can find an aerobic sport — or several of them — that you truly enjoy. Then it's no longer "I have to go exercise." It becomes, "Hey, I get to exercise today." Let's review some options:

Walking — This one is so easy to get into and so popular. Some walkers — mostly women — carry a weight in each hand in order to increase their heart rate. It's a great way to get a better workout. A weight vest, described earlier, can also raise your heart rate.

Running — This was the aerobics exercise of choice for many of us when we were in our twenties through forties, but senior runners are not as prevalent. The reason's pretty obvious. All of that pounding the pavement takes its toll on our bodies — feet, knees, hips and back, to name a few. Ted, now eighty-two, is an exception. He still runs five miles every other day and has no problems. It can be done.

Swimming — Is there an exercise that's easier on the body? Not only easier, but all of the body — arms, legs, trunk — gets a workout, plus it's easy to keep an elevated heart rate. Those of us with sciatica pain from a herniated disc quickly learned the virtues of swimming laps.

Swimming doesn't involve weight bearing, which is good for preventing stress on the joints, but it's not a good activity for strengthening bones. If you do a lot of swimming for fitness, include some walking or running activities as well as strength training to promote bone strength.

Cycling — It's easy on the body and easy to do. All you need is a decent bike, helmet and a few other essentials. Cycling with a group adds to the enjoyment. Some question cycling in traffic, a justifiable concern. Many get over it once they've done it for awhile, but others choose not to risk injury. You may find a bike path away from any highway near you. They're safer than roads with traffic.

Gyms — One of the great benefits of going to a gym is that you can vary your aerobics activity — treadmill, arc trainer, elliptical trainer, whatever. Variety can definitely increase enjoyment, plus it's good for the body to do different routines.

Classes — Many gyms offer classes that involve aerobic activity. They have the distinct advantage of involving others, becoming your impromptu support group. It's hard to stop exercising when the people around you are going full out. One of the best classes is spinning, which normally includes intervals.

Some gyms offer special classes designed to generate an aerobic and anaerobic workout. Examples are Cross-Fit, P90X and Boot Camp. P90X is also available via DVDs you can purchase so that it can be done at home. I have friends who've done each and speak very highly of them.

Cross-Country Skiing — This one is truly a winner. It works the upper and lower body and gets the heart pumping at a high rate quickly. If you have access to this sport in your region, by all means try it.

Canoeing and Kayaking — These are very enjoyable exercise but remember: you have to move, not just paddle occasionally. The same rules apply as in brisk walking versus a stroll. Brisk paddling will generate an aerobic workout.

CROSS-TRAINING

We are all creatures of habit. We get comfortable doing something and stick with it versus adding variety. We like the treadmill at the gym and use it every time, or the stationary bike or arc trainer. We get into a routine.

Our bodies get used to the routine, too, and find it more relaxing. More relaxation is not why we're there. We need to trick our bodies, use different muscles by doing different exercises. Variety also helps strengthen the circuits, synapses and neurons in the brain, as we covered earlier.

I cycle a lot in SW Florida in the winter and ride a cart while playing golf, a requirement. When I get back to Bucks County, PA, in May and started walking the golf course, carrying my bag, my legs hurt more than if I'd done a hard bike ride for four hours. Cycling muscles and walking muscles are not the same. This year I plan to do some brisk walking in Florida as well as cycling.

Break out of the mold. Use the treadmill one day, arc trainer the next. Your body will appreciate and respond to the variety.

MARC'S JOURNEY

Elizabeth I, the copy editor for my final manuscript, told me about the transformation of Marc J, her brother-in-law. Here's his story:

"In December 2008, four months before my sixtieth birthday, I had an opportunity to see my silhouette. My first thought was, 'I look like the opening of the old Alfred Hitchcock show.' It wasn't that I didn't know I was grossly overweight and horribly out of shape; of course I knew that. But the image set off a switch in my head and I declared to myself that something must be done!

"The first week of January 2009, I checked myself into Jenny Craig — I needed adult supervision. I set a weight loss goal of fifty pounds and committed to the diet. I began walking several times a week because that was all I could do. By the end of April I'd reached the halfway point on my diet and decided to run. By June I was running four days a week, but I knew I hadn't done any upper body or core work in eight years and I had to start something.

"I'd seen the P90X infomercials many times. I was a bit skeptical but figured I'd try it. When I received it I was too embarrassed to take the fit test, especially since I knew I would fail it. I started the program and followed the ninety schedule to the T. When I started I could barely do any of the moves and certainly not at the level of the people on the DVDs. But I persisted and finished the program. As promised, I made huge gains in muscle strength, cardio strength and flexibility, plus body fat loss.

"In August 2009, I reached my fifty-pound weight loss goal. When I finished P90X I did the full P90Xplus program while I continued to run. My knees were bothering me, so I sought a cardio alternative. I found a cardio program from the same company that makes P90X called "Insanity." I did that program four times and then did another of their cardio programs called "Insanity, The Asylum." I think I'm the oldest person in America to have completed that program.

"I've maintained my weight for two years while gaining lots of muscles. My cardio is excellent and I was able to get off my type 2 diabetes medications.

"I communicate with a lot of people over fifty, some over sixty, who've done these programs. Age is no barrier to fitness."

LET'S REVIEW

- Exercising aerobically at sixty percent to seventy percent or Zone 1 is a big deal. This level burns fat and gets your cardiovascular system functioning at a good level. Even elite athletes spend most of their exercise time in this zone.

- Once you've taken the training wheels off, spending some time in your anaerobic zone — that's eighty percent or more or Zone 3, depending on your conditioning, which determines your AT (anaerobic threshold) — is also a big deal. Your metabolism goes up, you burn more calories afterward and your cardiovascular system gets even stronger. Remember that the more intense the exercise the more calories you'll burn during and after the activity.

- Information is a good thing. If you're a walker, get a pedometer. See how many steps you're really doing — but this won't tell you how hard you're working. Whatever your exercise activity, buy a heart rate monitor, one that provides information that will motivate you.

- Find others to do exercise with you. It can make a big difference in your consistency and enjoyment. Showing up is a huge deal, the difference between success and failure.

- Find one or more activities that you truly enjoy doing.

- It takes time for a new activity to become a habit. Stick with it until that happens, no matter what. Make it your job; not a temporary job but a permanent one. If you waiver, remember your reasons for doing this in the first place.

GLASBERGEN

**"Weight lifting can help lower your cholesterol.
Load up your fork with veggies and lift it
to your mouth. Do 3 sets of 15 reps daily."**

CHAPTER SIX — STRENGTH TRAINING

"Eighty percent of success is showing up." — *Woody Allen*

HERE'S WHAT'S COMING

- Why is it important to do strength training?

- Why do it "to fatigue," and what does that mean?

- What are slow-twitch and fast-twitch muscles and why should you care?

- How do you avoid hurting yourself?

- How much is enough?

- What's the difference between concentri c and eccentric? Is it important?

- What if you don't have time or access to a gym?

- What's so important about writing down what you do?

- Should a woman worry about getting muscle bound?

The following quote is from Leo Tolstoy, 1897:
"The most difficult subjects can be explained to the most slow-witted man if he has not formed any idea of them already. But the simplest thing cannot be made clear to the most intelligent man if he is firmly persuaded that he knows already, without a shadow of doubt, what is laid before him."

How does this relate to strength training? I've watched friends at our gym exercising with weights and occasionally have asked them what their goals are. I've received answers like "improve muscle tone," "improve my coordination" and "retain flexibility." These are all valid objectives.

Additional goals could/should be to "build stronger muscles, bones, ligaments and tendons so that I can remain strong and independent into my old age." Unfortunately, many individuals undertaking strength training exercises aren't working hard enough to make these goals a reality.

Many don't believe it when informed that they should be working harder — sometimes much harder. As one friend said recently, "That goes against everything I've ever learned." What he didn't say is that what he learned was forty years ago. Another friend said, after reading the strength training recommendations of a noted gerontologist, "Seniors should not be doing strength training to fatigue; that's it. I don't want to talk about it anymore."

In this chapter we'll discuss what you need to do to build strength and maintain your independence into your old age. We're going to talk about doing strength training to fatigue. We'll explain what "to fatigue" means — that's important to understand. It may sound a bit scary if you've never done it, but we're going to begin in the wading pool and work up to the deep end gradually. We won't suggest that you do exercise that'll lead to injury. We're going to begin by working at where you are, not where you'll be in six months. You'll begin working at a comfortable weight level and increase it gradually as you get stronger. You will get stronger.

Muscle enlargement is called **hypertrophy**. When we exercise a muscle to the point where we can't do any more repetitions this acts as a catalyst within the muscle fibers (cells) to build up more muscle proteins, which are responsible for muscle contraction. Over repeated exercise sessions the muscle increases its ability to lift heavier weights and also enlarges.

"To fatigue" means doing an exercise until you can't do more while maintaining proper form. It doesn't involve yanking, jerking and getting into contortions to

move weight that you otherwise couldn't lift.

As a result of repeated, exhaustive stimulation, muscle fibers undergo a number of important changes at the cellular level. The net effect is an enlargement or hypertrophy of the stimulated muscle. The number of muscle fibers doesn't change, but the muscle as a whole enlarges because each muscle fiber increases in diameter. A champion weight lifter or body builder is an excellent example of hypertrophy. Don't worry, there's no chance that you'll go there.

Men may remember when they were in high school gym class and were asked to do as many pushups as they could. When they could do no more they stopped. Their triceps and chest muscles gave all they had. *Those particular muscles were "fatigued," not their entire body. That's what "to fatigue" means.*

Remember the story in the last chapter about Neale and Ned climbing Mt. Washington? We aren't talking about that kind of fatigue, where they felt like they couldn't take another step.

Strength training to fatigue means you expand that idea to other muscle groups such as your legs, back, biceps, etc. You need to rest a day or two after pushing your muscles for the repair and rebuild process to work. Twice a week is fine; you can do three times, but no more.

Some of us lifted weights when we were younger. The name of the game then was to lift more than our friends to show how strong we were. That's not the game today. The goal now — for both men and women — is to help us become the best we can be today, independent of anyone else. This is a personal best, not competition best.

Serious athletes — those playing competitive sports at a high level — have recognized the value of strength training for many years. It's only in the last twenty years or so that some of the rest of us have learned this as a result of research done by those studying aging.

A ROSE BY ANY OTHER NAME

There are three phrases used to describe proper strength training: to exhaustion, to fatigue or to failure. All three mean the same thing — lifting a weight until you can't do another repetition while using proper form. The goal should be eight to twelve repetitions. If you can do more it's time to increase the weight.

I've used the term "to fatigue" as it's the one that I think has a "kinder, gentler" tone to it. You'll encounter the use of "to exhaustion" frequently in books and articles. I've found that many people misinterpret "to exhaustion." They think it means their whole body is exhausted.

ABOUT MUSCLE AND BONE LOSS

We all know that **osteoporosis** is the loss of bone mass due to age. My mother had it. She fell and broke her hip as a result and never recovered. There are many similar stories.

Ever heard of **sarcopenia**? It's the loss of muscle mass and function, also due to age. It's a good word, has a nice sound to it, but it's definitely not good news when it happens. Beginning in our thirties or early forties most of us lose about a quarter pound of muscle per year. Multiply that by twenty or thirty years and we're talking lots of muscle loss.

The bad news, of course, is that osteoporosis and sarcopenia happen to all of us as we age and there's little we can do about it, right? You say no? You know that we can take calcium pills daily and reduce the bone loss, right? Well, the calcium may help if your diet is very deficient in calcium. But the effectiveness of calcium supplements is limited. Most effective is the calcium supplement *and* engagement in weight-bearing exercise, as this promotes calcium deposition into bones, making them stronger.

Let's get back to sarcopenia. That's just nature at work. It is what it is. There's little we can do about it, right? Wrong. Sarcopenia, by the way, is even more prevalent as we age than osteoporosis.

The key to slowing down sarcopenia is a consistent exercise program involving both aerobic and strength training activities. Aerobics improves respiratory capacity, blood flow and aids the process of storing glycogen in muscle cells. This provides the energy we need for daily life and exercise. Strength training improves bone density, muscle mass, stability and balance.

THE FACTS

About ten percent of muscle mass is lost from age twenty-five to fifty years. Then, from age fifty to eighty years, another 40 percent is lost. This means a total of fifty percent of muscle mass is lost by age eighty.

Skeletal muscle fibers become smaller in diameter. The result is a reduction in muscle strength and endurance and a tendency to fatigue more rapidly. Because cardiovascular performance also decreases with age, blood flow to active muscles doesn't increase with exercise as rapidly as it does in younger people.

Aging skeletal muscles develop increasing amounts of fibrous connective tissue, a process called fibrosis. Fibrosis makes the muscle less flexible and the collagen fibers can restrict movement and circulation.

Tolerance for exercise decreases. A lower tolerance for exercise results in part from the tendency for more rapid fatigue and part from the reduction in the ability to eliminate the heat generated during muscular contraction.

The ability to recover from muscular injuries decreases. The number of certain types of cells steadily decreases with age and the amount of fibrous tissue increases. When an injury occurs, repair capabilities are limited and scar tissue formation is the usual result.

While the muscular guy, now in his sixties, who used to hit his golf drives 250 yards and today can only hit it 200 yards is unhappy, his is not the biggest problem. Think about the men or women who started with little and now have almost nothing. Their opportunities to enjoy physical activity are greatly diminished and their chances of injury are now off the charts.

Now to the good news: *muscle mass can, for the most part, be retained and even increased by a consistent strength-training program.* A progressive strength-training program has produced very large gains in strength training even for those in their nineties.

In one study Ben Hurley of the University of Maryland recruited twenty-three healthy men and women in their sixties and seventies to implement strength training for only one of their legs three times a week. In nine weeks the exercised leg increased in muscle size by twelve percent and in strength by thirty percent. Let's hope they worked on the other leg for the next nine weeks.

A SENSE OF WHERE YOU ARE

Here's another term — **proprioception**. This is the ability to sense the position, location, orientation and movement of the body and its parts. Proprioception enables us to know where we are and what we want to do without having to think about it. Proprioception is dramatically improved by a complete exercise program.

In 1999, John McPhee published a revised edition of his book, *A Sense of Where You Are: Bill Bradley at Princeton*. The first edition of the book was published when Bradley was a student at Princeton in the mid-1960s.

It's the story of Bradley as a basketball star at Princeton and a Rhodes Scholar at Oxford. He went on to play in the NBA and then became a U.S. Senator. The title came from the fact that Bradley could sink basketball shots from all over the court without ever looking at the basket. He told McPhee that after many hundreds of hours of practice you develop "A sense of where you are."

We can walk, run, jump, throw a ball, climb stairs and do many other things without ever thinking about them. Imagine what life would be like if we had to think before every move. These abilities are due to the magic of that big word: proprioception. Aerobics and strength training are important ingredients in our ability to maintain proprioception as we age. These activities help prevent falls, a big issue as we get older, because we don't "bounce" the way we used to.

EXERCISE AND NURSING HOMES

Bob has been my urologist for years. He's a delightful guy, now seventy. He loves his work and says he will retire when he no longer enjoys his profession. During my last visit I mentioned that I was writing this book. He was pleased to hear it as he's very supportive of exercise, including his own.

He told me about his mother-in-law, who had to go into a nursing home at age eighty-two due to health issues. This home required that all residents participate in daily exercise programs, something she'd never done. She didn't have a history of doing any exercise. Whether it was good genes, the exercise, or both, the result was that she lived to ninety-seven, never had a broken bone and was mentally and physically alert to the end.

Is it ever too late to start an exercise program? Ninety-year-olds have doubled their leg strength with three months of regular exercise.

SLOW AND FAST — WE NEED BOTH

All muscle fibers are mainly comprised of two types, Type I, slow-twitch, and Type II, fast-twitch; they're intermingled within our muscles.

Slow-twitch fibers are able to contract repeatedly without much fatigue. Slow-twitch muscle fibers have a high aerobic capacity, meaning they can produce energy for a long time provided sufficient oxygen is available. The ability to go on a long walk or bike ride requires lots of slow-twitch muscles.

Fast-twitch fibers have a high anaerobic capacity — they can produce power without oxygen for a relatively short period of time. Sprinters have lots of fast-twitch muscle fibers because they're executing short-term, intense activity using stored muscle sugar (glycogen).

We're all born with a fixed percentage of slow-twitch and fast-twitch muscle fibers. Across a broad population, muscle composition is forty percent to fifty percent Type I, and fifty percent to sixty percent Type II. To some extent we can change these proportions. Endurance exercise will decrease the proportion of Type II and increase proportion of Type I, but there's less evidence demonstrating changing Type I to Type II. Our physical activities determine what happens, including increasing muscle mass and strength by engaging in activity, or losing mass and strength due to inactivity.

We lose more fast-twitch muscle fibers than we do slow-twitch muscle fibers as we age simply because we don't use them enough. We need the fast-twitch fibers for golf, lifting weights, accelerating while cycling or running. Slow-twitch fibers are for endurance; long cycling trips, hiking or walking. The loss of fast-twitch muscle fibers due to lack of use is why golfers complain about not being able to hit the ball as far as they used to. Strength training is the best way to activate the underused fast-twitch muscle fibers.

An increase in muscle mass in response to muscle use is called muscle hypertrophy. It's the opposite of muscle atrophy, which results from muscle inactivity and aging. Usually both occur simultaneously. The good news with aging loss is that the loss is not as great in older individuals as it is in younger individuals because there is less to lose. The bad news is that reversing this in older individuals is more difficult. It takes longer to produce hypertrophy, but it can be done.

HELP ME UP

The comments section following an article in *The New York Times* on muscle loss had some interesting statements. One responder said he attended a lecture at his YMCA on aging and was shocked to learn that his daily twelve-mile bike ride and a weekly yoga session did not address the main culprit of muscle wasting — fast-twitch muscle fibers. He didn't realize fast-twitch muscles are needed for balance and hence quality of life.

As a result he started a twice-a-week strength-training program. He was motivated by what the lecturer said: "Do it if you want to delay having someone having to help you off the toilet."

A FORMULA FOR STRENGTH TRAINING

- Hire a trainer. This can be an excellent use of resources. View a trainer as an investment in your health, similar to a financial advisor for financial issues. Learn how to execute strength training properly, through a complete range of motion. Check in again two months later if not sooner and make some changes to your program so that your body continues to be challenged. Some use a trainer not only for technical assistance but also to provide encouragement and motivation.

- If spending money for a trainer is an issue, buy one or more books on strength training, make a list of exercises and then go do them. I'll list some books at the end of this book that are excellent. Take a book with you to the gym so that you can review the pictures and instructions before executing the exercise. Using proper form — doing an exercise correctly — is very important. Poor form can lead to injury, which can lead to giving up.

- Begin with light weights or work on weight machines versus dumbbells or barbells. Get your muscles used to the process; don't overload them. If you're sore, wait until the soreness goes away. You're in a marathon, not a sprint.

- Be sure to warm up your body. Hop on a treadmill, exercise bike or whatever for ten minutes or more and then do some stretching exercises involving your back and stomach muscles, legs and arms at the end. Take the time to cool down at the end. Both are good physically and mentally plus help make the "work" of strength training more enjoyable.

- Leave sufficient time for all of these activities. Stretching at the end will reduce muscle tension and the potential for later muscle use strain.

- After doing lighter weight exercises for a few months, gradually increase the weights used. Then move to lifting weights to fatigue — lifting or pushing the weights until you can't move them. Do two sets of eight to twelve reps, and once you're there, do this type of exercise at *least twice a week for the rest of your life.* As your strength increases you can gradually increase the resistance — the amount of weight you lift.

- In order to progress and gain you must incorporate the principle of **overload.** This is the process of progressively increasing the resistance which will increase the gains. If you reach a certain point and level off you'll not show any further improvement in strength.

- If you level off and don't increase resistance but continue to work out you'll retain what you have and resist both osteoporosis and sarcopenia.

Harry Truman said, "There's nothing new except the history you don't know." That's true about the principle of overload; the first application was by an Olympic wrestler, Milo of Cortona, in 500 BC. He started carrying a bull calf on his back each day until the calf was fully grown.

TWO CONFESSIONS

You've now read about the value of hiring a trainer. Remember the story of the shoemaker's kids? That's me. I consciously or subconsciously thought, "I'm writing a book about this. I know a lot, so I don't really need some trainer telling me what to do. I might even know more than they do — they should come to me." *I was wrong. It's painful to admit but true — in spades.*

As part of a special program we're running at our fitness center in SW Florida I had an hour with Stacey, one of the trainers. Stacey is a happy, smiling, enthusiastic individual perfectly suited for her job.

My problem was that I'd been doing many of the same exercises for years. I liked them and enjoyed doing them, but they weren't doing much for me. My brain told my muscles, "He's going to do the same thing he did last week and the week before and the week before that. We can just relax and take a nap." You don't build new synapses in the brain by doing this; you just maintain what you already have.

In addition, my stretching routines had gone south. I had gotten out of the habit of doing a variety of stretching after my workout and was down to just a couple during the workout. Why, you say? I have no excuse that will have any legitimacy.

Stacey quickly got me doing new exercises that required my muscles to fire in different ways. I also had to concentrate on what I was doing versus just daydreaming while doing the same old thing. What a difference. I left an hour later more tired than I'd been after a workout in a long time.

I plan to have a session with Stacey once a week for at least a month. I want to be sure that I really understand how to do these exercises properly, not just close to properly. That takes repetition and concentration along with coaching. I also plan to meet with her again in eight weeks or sooner so that we can revise the program again.

I sent this to Art, who has a regular and rigorous exercise program and he responded:

"I like it, and interestingly enough I came to a similar conclusion about myself yesterday. I have two basic workouts in the gym that I alternate, one a cardio and the other strength building. I made very rapid progress for three months but lately the progress is minimal, and for the first time yesterday I felt bored by the gym and didn't want to go through the pain. I did, but resolved to get a trainer later this week to get a new perspective. I keep my gym time short and intense, usually about an hour and fifteen minutes, and when I leave I'm fried, either from aerobics or weights."

FOR MEN ONLY

I am not now nor have I ever been a gymnast. Suppose a gymnast enticed me into his playground and said, "Harry, I'm going to put this eight-foot balance beam a foot off the ground. It's the six-inch-wide model for beginners like you.

What I'd like you to do is walk across it, forwards and backwards." I think I could do that, no problem.

Suppose he said, "Harry, to make it more interesting we're going to move the beam up to five feet off the ground. And, to add to the challenge, we're going to put it on top of that concrete slab over there. Now I'd like you to just walk across it going forward and backwards."

I'd say something like, "Man, are you crazy? There is no way I'm getting on that bar at that height over that slab!" He didn't change the task but he did change the risk. The same applies for strength training.

Men sometimes have a need or desire to do dumb things in the interest of proving their manhood. This may also apply to some women, though none I know. When you first go to the gym and see somebody you know or even somebody you don't know lifting weights to fatigue — don't go there.

If you do, the result, at minimum, will be very sore muscles. More likely you'll do serious damage to some muscles, ligaments or tendons and end up not being able to work out for a long time. You may even decide that strength training isn't your cup of tea. Be smart about it. Be patient and use common sense. Start slowly, don't strain yourself and build up to heavier weight gradually.

FOR WOMEN ONLY

Strength training has been found to be beneficial for women who've survived breast cancer but have lymphedema — fluid retention and tissue swelling in the lymphatic system. Women who implemented a slow, progressive strength-training program had fewer problems than women who didn't do strength training. Gretchen Reynolds wrote about this in *The New York Times* article "Phys. Ed: Lifting Weights After Breast Cancer" on December 22, 2010.

In the same article she said, "Another study released this month suggests that progressive weight training in older women can confer significant and lasting benefits on mental and physical conditioning." A study she quotes reported that women who had lifted weights once a week had better cognitive function and suffered thirty percent fewer falls than a control group who only did toning and stretching.

LEARN FROM THE PROS

One of the reasons we watch individual sports like golf and tennis on television is to learn from the pros — the men and women who really know what they're doing. We hope to have some "monkey-see, monkey-do" results.

While your gym may not have professionals, every gym has men and women exercising who clearly know what they're doing. A friend told me how he chooses exercises; "I watch the good guys and do what they do." It's OK to even ask them about it. Most are happy to help and, if asked politely, will be flattered.

LIFTING TO WHAT?

Lifting weights to fatigue is when you're using the correct form and can't physically lift or push a weight another time. This damages muscle cells — not the muscles but the cells, and they grow back stronger. Muscle cells need time to recover, so don't do strength training daily.

You'll recover quickly after lifting a weight to fatigue, in terms of being able to do another set of exercises or other activities, but your body will need time to construct the new cellular tissue. You need to rest those muscles for a day or two after pushing your muscles for the repair and rebuilding process to work. Twice-a-week workouts are fine. You can do three times, but no more.

The reasons to do strength training to fatigue are to benefit from having stronger muscles, bones, ligaments and tendons, and to achieve greater speed and endurance. It also helps the nerves that control coordination and balance. It'll help you stay active and independent well into an advanced old age. And you'll not only feel better, you'll look better too.

Weight training is particularly beneficial to fast-twitch muscles, those explosive ones. Yes, with increased strength you may be able to hit the little white ball — or fuzzy yellow ball — farther. That alone may be a good enough reason to do it.

Remember: you don't **start** a strength-training program by lifting weights to fatigue, not even close. Begin easy, using light weights and machines. Work up to heavier weights over a period of several months, not a few days. A good trainer will get you started properly. Keeping records, which we'll discuss soon, will motivate you to work harder.

Here's a suggestion that may make resistance training more palatable and productive:

- Instead of trying to do everything every visit, pick some body parts to work on one day and then others on the next visit. For example, you might do legs, core and chest on Tuesday and then back and arms on Thursday. If you do two sets of eight to twelve reps to fatigue for a series of exercises, you've done enough. Your core incorporates the muscles of your stomach and lower back.

- Use the proper form. If you exercise incorrectly you could hurt your body, especially as you approach the fatigue stage. Form counts.

- Do big muscle groups first; quadriceps, then hamstrings and calves.

What if you're a woman — can you get big muscles? It's not likely since you don't have the necessary testosterone for it — unless you take steroids. If you see some competitive women weight lifters with big muscles it's likely they're on steroids, whether they admit it or not. Women have about ten percent of the testosterone of men. What will happen is you'll get stronger and have more muscle definition.

THE QUESTION

"OK, Harry, you've made your point. Doing strength training to fatigue is a good idea. It's the way to get maximum results. However — and this is a big however — I just don't think I'm ready or willing to work that hard. I've done some strength training over the years — light to medium weights, couple of sets, ten to fifteen reps each — and maybe I'll go back to doing that. But lifting weights to fatigue — I don't think so. What if I just do some light or medium lifting — am I doing any good?"

THE ANSWER

Is something better than nothing? Do you receive some benefit even if you don't work that hard? The answer is yes. You're putting some minor strain on muscles and ligaments plus helping flexibility and coordination. You'll derive some measure of benefit, clearly more than if you did nothing.

And maybe, just maybe, if you do something for a few months or longer, one day you'll say, "Self, this is not all that hard, and I have the time. Why don't I try doing what Harry suggested and work a bit harder? And, if that feels OK, maybe I'll try that "to fatigue" and see how I feel after a few weeks. If I do it gradually I shouldn't run any risk of pulling a muscle and missing out on all the fun things I like to do. And maybe it will even make all those enjoyable activities even more fun."

EINSTEIN AND INSANITY

You've likely heard Einstein's definition of insanity; "Doing the same thing over and over again and expecting different results." Once you've done a series of exercises for a few months your body gets used to doing them. The hippocampus section of the brain says to the muscles, "We've been here lots of times now. We can do these exercises with our eyes closed, no sweat. We don't even have to work that hard."

You need to vary your routine so that your brain and muscles do things they're not comfortable with. That maximizes results for time spent, which is one of our goals. George said, "It reminded me of what my first trainer told me — the key to a good investment strategy is diversification. It's also the key to a good exercise program. Changing your routine makes it less boring and more effective."

A friend has been doing a program called Crossfit for some months now. He works out with a small group two or three times a week, very intense. They never do the same exercises two days in a row. They're constantly "tricking" the body by doing new exercises. Mark loves it and says it's had a dramatic impact on his fitness, endurance and energy.

TAKE A BREAK

Neale said: "I'm not sure if you will agree with this, but in my experience it helps to throw in a very easy week every six or eight weeks. Don't stop working out altogether, just do a very light version of your routine to give your body a chance to really recover. This is especially important for those new to the concept of working out really hard. These people tend to overdo things, and that's likely to induce injuries that slow you down for months."

Good suggestion, Neale, and one well worth following. It becomes more important the older we get.

KATHY'S PROGRAM

Kathy, now fifty, has two young kids and has been doing strength training regularly for thirty years. She said:

"I had some initial thoughts about not stressing the need to always do two sets to exhaustion because some people may not be able to find the time, motivation or focus to always adhere to this approach. As my life demands have changed my rule of thumb is always to do strength training two to three times per week no matter how much time I have — and to always do at least the core work *very hard*. I think the intensity is the key thing.

"For example, I'm always very pressed for time when I get to the gym at 5:30 AM in order to get home by 6:20 AM for Alex's school bus. So I do maximum weight to fatigue for one set of twelve to fourteen reps. I still feel the workout, even if it's not two sets.

"One tremendous benefit of continually lifting weights since age twenty is that at age fifty I look just as good in a tank top as I did thirty years ago, not to mention wearing smaller jeans than I did in college. That's something to smile about!"

CONCENTRIC AND ECCENTRIC — A BIG DEAL

All males love to have big biceps. They are not the most important muscles to have by any means, but they look so good. Men admire other men who have big ones.

Suppose you go to your gym and decide to do some bicep curls. You pick a weight that you can curl eight to twelve times and go at it. Most of us emphasize the raising of the weight when we curl our arm, which contracts the muscle. This is a concentric contraction. We then quickly lower it.

Instead of lowering it quickly, lower it very slowly. Try to do a count of two on the way up and a count of four on the way down. The lowering of the weight is an eccentric contraction, in which the force is resisted as the muscle lengthens. And guess what — adding the eccentric muscle work generates more muscle strength than just the concentric contractions.

Here's how it works: when you do concentric contraction the muscle shortens through the range of movement. The shorter the muscle is relative to itself, the less force that can be generated and the less movement that can occur.

As you lower the weight slowly, the muscle doing the work is lengthening — an eccentric contraction — and the additional force generated enables you to control the weight. This also makes the muscle work harder and it builds more tissue.

To prove this to yourself, try the following experiment. Curl your usual weight until you can't produce maximum elbow flexion; the muscle is "fatigued." Then lower the weight slowly and hold it in a new position until you no longer can maintain the position. You've fatigued the muscle again.

At this stage try to curl back to the last position; it's impossible to do. But you can lower the weight slowly to a new position by eccentric contraction and hold the new position. If you do this you will get a better workout, doing the same number of curls as before.

This applies to all strength training, not just bicep curls. Try it with the strength training exercises you do. Talk to your trainer and ask him or her to watch you to be sure you're doing it correctly.

MORE IS BETTER

Exercise physiologists have examined lots of data and concluded that multiple sets versus a single set are more effective at improving strength over time. They also suggest that fewer reps with heavier weights trump more reps with lighter weights. The former builds muscle while the latter builds endurance.

How many reps should you do? Many studies suggest eight to twelve per set. One reputable book suggested that older adults use slightly lighter weights and do ten to fifteen. My senior friends who do serious strength training generally do eight to twelve, as do I.

GYMS AND TRAINERS

The first trip to a gym can be intimidating. It seems like everyone — except you — knows exactly what he or she is doing. Maybe you can see some people working out who are slim, trim, sweating and hard at work. You'll also see some people working out who are not slim or trim who are sweating and hard at work. When you first walk into a gym go up to the desk, introduce yourself and say something like, "I'm new at this and I need your help." You'll get it, guaranteed.

How do you go about selecting a trainer? How do you know a good one from a mediocre or poor one? Good questions. You're not looking for a new best friend, nor should your trainer be. Sharing your life's secrets is not the reason for being there. A male should not pick the most gorgeous female trainer any more than a female should select the hot male hunk. At least that shouldn't be your primary reason for picking them. You'd like someone who is cordial, clear in his or her directions, encouraging, knowledgeable and who understands your goals.

A good trainer will make an assessment of your current physical condition as part of the first session. He or she will also ask about your goals and then will develop a program with you tailored to your needs. The program should be results driven.

What do you do if you and the trainer don't connect? The same thing you'd do with a doctor, hair stylist, dentist or anyone else providing personal service — find someone else. You're the client and you decide. Make no mistake — the relationship you have with your trainer is critical. He or she can be your mini-support group.

How often should you use a trainer? Some need one every time to provide support; they may also provide motivation to show up. Others like a monthly checkup to be sure they're on target. *The minimum is every two months for a checkup and to make changes in your routine so that your body doesn't go on automatic pilot.*

Consider sharing a trainer with a partner — your spouse or a friend. Then you can go to the gym together, work to keep each other using good form, working hard and, most importantly, showing up. Your partner may even offer good suggestions since you both are learning from the same trainer.

Would you like to avoid injury? A trainer will teach you the right way to do exercises so that you don't hurt yourself.

HALYNA'S TRAINER

An example from Halyna: "My own personal story about working with a trainer: I have pooh-poohed the notion for years, saying I know what I need to do, I am reasonably physically fit, I can't afford a trainer, that's for people who aren't motivated, don't know what they're doing, etc.

"Well, you convinced me to try it (even though when Bill tried to talk me into it, I said no), and I've had five sessions and consider it money well spent — I'm doing strength training I would never have gotten into on my own. I'm taking a break from the trainer now and then will go back to her on a monthly basis."

NO GYM OR NO TIME

Suppose you don't have easy access to a gym or the time to go. Do you have an option?

Sure you do — work out at home, primarily using your own body weight to produce results. There are lots of exercises you can do without any equipment. Many of these and other exercises can be done to fatigue without any equipment. Examples:

- Push-ups

- Stomach crunches

- Arm dips between two chairs

- Side plank crunches — lie on your side on your elbow and bend your body toward the floor

- Chin-ups – rig a bar in a doorway

- Walking lunges — good for warm-up

How about purchasing a few items that will increase your options? Some examples and their approximate cost:

- Exercise ball or Fitball — $40

- Bosu Ball — $120

- Exercise bands — They vary in resistance, under $10 each

- Dual grip exercise ball — $60

- Chin-up bar for doorway — $40

An interesting option that's being used now by a number of gyms is the TRX Suspension Training System. This system can be attached to any door and provides the opportunity for up to 300 exercises. You can acquire this system for about $200. Check fitnessanywhere.com. You can even take the TRX straps and a few exercise bands with you when you travel so that you can work out in your hotel room.

Whatever you do — be sure you're properly executing the exercises you choose.

ONLINE OPTIONS

The *Wall Street Journal* published an article by Alina Dizik, "Feel the Burn (Not the Shame) of a Workout Class." It summarized the features and benefits of several websites that offer online classes. Three of them are archived and can be downloaded and one is live via webcam. The cost is per month or per class, depending on the site.

Ms. Dizik summarized: "Overall, the online classes were less boring than watching an exercise DVD and are a great option for those days when you can't get to the gym. Instructor quality was good and classes were easy to follow." A list of websites is at the end of this chapter.

TOM — THE ARTIFICIAL MAN

Tom played football at the University of Minnesota and was the MVP of the 1959 team. He also was a three-year starter for the Gophers baseball team, which won the National Championship in 1960. Physical contact and injuries during his college years led to problems:

Both shoulders replaced with artificial parts; left hip replacement; right big toe fusion; elbow and knee surgeries, plus two back surgeries; and a heart condition that required a stent in a serious place, called the "Widow Maker" artery. None of this is obvious when you look at him today. He's trim, the picture of fitness. But, you say, he needs to restrict his physical activity, given his history? Not a chance.

Tom does serious strength training three days a week. *By serious I mean he is lifting the heaviest weights he can for three sets of eight to ten reps.* He works a lot on his shoulders in order to build up the muscles around the artificial joints. He also does five days per week of cardio work, primarily on the treadmill — as much as he can as long as he can. This doesn't count four days of golf each week. Don't ask me how he does all of this — I have no idea.

After the stent was installed he asked his cardiologist whether he should continue his regimen. His doctor said, "Tom, when you get off the treadmill I want you to be crawling. The more you can do the better." He also supported his strength-training program.

Tom's physical problems are due to his strenuous, competitive activities as a young man. *The fact that he is alive, healthy, physically active and fit is a direct result of his exercise regimen today.*

WRITE IT DOWN

Years ago a sales trainer said, "Ninety-five percent of sales reps hate to make cold calls and the other five percent lie about it." The truth is that some of us who exercise lie about how much we do, even to ourselves. We don't write it down, so who knows whether we did one set or two, or how many reps? We conveniently forget and, as a result, miscount the total.

Very few men or women at our fitness center write down what they do, maybe one in ten. How do they know if they're getting better? If they do different exercises on different days, how do they keep track?

Keeping records in fitness is a big deal — and so easy to do. Not only does it keep us honest but there's that wonderful sense of satisfaction in seeing how much we've done and where we're getting better.

Use a spreadsheet or notepad for gym work. Many gyms will provide you with a form designed for this purpose. Check off the exercises you're going to do that day and then record the number of sets and reps. If the exercise involves weights, have a record of what weight you're using in a separate column and change it when the weight used changes.

Keep another record summarizing walking, swimming, running or cycling — distance, total time, average speed, time in various heart rate zones, even calories burned. A good heart rate monitor provides all of this information. Seeing progress over time is motivational, and motivation is a big deal. It keeps us going even on days that are less than optimal.

What if you're just starting out and only do a few exercises? You can easily remember what weight you're using and how many sets and reps you've done — do you really have to write it down? Probably not, but why not do it at the beginning so that when you've added exercises, maybe up to a total of ten or more, you're already in the habit?

GOLF AND STRENGTH TRAINING

The 1970s, 1980s and 1990s produced a lot of terrific golf instructors: Bob Toski, Paul Runyan, Davis Love Jr., David Leadbetter, Peter Kostis, Jim McLean and many more. They made a huge contribution to the abilities of professional and amateur golfers. It seems like all of them were negative on strength training for golfers.

I remember into the nineties hearing something like the following on television: "Strength training is bad for golfers. It'll make you muscle bound and restrict your ability to swing a club." If you looked at most of the pros of those years their heeding that advice is evident. Soft bellies and no real muscle tone were the norm.

An exception was that diminutive guy from South Africa, Gary Player, who marched to his own drummer. He won all of the majors, the Masters and British Open three times each and won over eighty times worldwide. He even won a Champions Tour event when he was in his sixties. He turns seventy-five this year and still competes occasionally. He was quoted in 2011, in the *Wall Street Journal*: "People said weight training was detrimental to golfers. I was squatting 325 pounds the night before I won the U.S. Open in 1965. Today the players have traveling gyms." Arnold Palmer was also fit in his prime, as was Greg Norman, who came along later.

And then, along came Tiger Woods in 1996. In short order he went from the scrawny kid who could hit the ball a mile to the muscular man who could hit it a mile and a half. He changed the rules of exercise for golfers as well as other elements of golf; a new paradigm.

Take note of the athleticism of the young guys on tour. A good example — one of many — is Camilo Villegas; he's rippling with muscles. He's so athletic that an announcer mentioned recently that he could make the Columbia cycling team. Or Paul Casey — ever look at his forearms?

The Masters Par Three Contest was televised last spring and Palmer, Player and Nicklaus were playing together. Unfortunately, only one of the three was fit; you know which one.

WHAT ABOUT GAINING WEIGHT?

Some more good news: Muscle mass takes up less space than fat and burns more calories. You end up with an improved body shape, better muscle tone and more functional strength. Muscle weighs more than fat. You may lose fat, gain muscle and not be any lighter in pounds. In fact, you may even weigh more, but you sure won't look or feel like the old you.

The basal rate of fat metabolism is about five calories per pound compared to ten to twenty calories per pound of muscle mass. As you increase muscle and decrease fat your BMR (basal metabolic rate) will increase. A study at Tufts University of men and women who took up strength training three days a week showed that they increased their BMR by fifteen percent. They were burning 200 to 300 more calories every day.

Remember that to achieve these results you must lift enough weight to stimulate muscle growth. Just lifting a light weight twenty times won't do it. That's why building up over time to working to fatigue is important. This is a huge benefit because it means you can limit dieting and calorie restriction. You can get out and do more because you are stronger and more fit. You can go home and enjoy the "fruits" of your labor with a good meal.

WHAT'S DIFFERENT FOR WOMEN?

You have about ten percent of the testosterone of men; this is the primary source of larger muscles for males. As a result, your chances of getting big muscles are limited.

You'll gain all of the benefits that males do, like strength, less body fat, nice muscle definition, stronger bones, better athletic performance, reduction in the risk of injuries and back problems plus improved health.

Think about it — whatever sport you enjoy, whether it's golf, tennis, cycling, skiing — you'll be able to do it better. Golfers who do strength training can hit the ball farther; cyclists can cycle longer and faster without getting fatigued. Skiers are less likely to suffer injury when they fall.

Another big one is osteoporosis. You increase bone density significantly via strength training. You'll also reduce your risk of heart disease and diabetes. All of these are huge.

Why don't more women do strength training? I don't know; I suspect much of it is due to a lack of understanding of the benefits and a misconception that they can get "muscle bound." Even women in their seventies and eighties have significantly improved their strength by implementing a strength-training program. Women at this age should definitely hire a trainer to work with them and develop a program suitable to their individual ability.

VIEWS OF TWO WOMEN

Pat, a woman in her fifties, said: "Strength training is so very important for all the reasons you described. A few other benefits that I've found that you didn't mention:

"Better posture — helps reverse the stoop of older age. Better posture leads to a more confident look and feel.

"It helps reverse or delay the sagging that occurs with age. The physical improvement is noticeable. I've been surprised by the change in my body over the last two years of doing only two to three strength classes per week. I look fitter and feel better than ever. My arms, legs, waist are all more toned than ever. It really helps.

"You are stronger — can do other things in your daily life that are important — climbing stairs, carrying groceries, doing household chores."

Kathy, also in her fifties, added:

"I believe that the key to maintaining my weight, low BMI and good posture/muscle tone has been thirty years of weight lifting. Very few of my friends in their fifties continue to lift weights and they wonder why their triceps start flapping in the breeze under their arms!"

READY, FIRE, AIM

Men tend to start an exercise program without spending much time planning what they're going to do, while women tend to want to think about it to develop a detailed plan before getting started. This is according to several articles I've read.

They can learn from each other. A plan is a good idea, but getting started is also. Delaying until everything is just perfect is not a good plan. Try a bit of both by getting going and doing something — walk, jog, cycle, stretch, whatever. When you have a bit of momentum, develop a plan for your daily and weekly exercise activities.

THE MIRACLE OF COMPOUNDING

Remember when we could earn six percent on a CD or is that too long ago to recall? If you could earn that today a $1,000 investment would double in twelve years; the miracle of compound interest — earning interest on interest is the key.

Let's apply that to building muscle mass. As you exercise you use a lot of fat as your energy source and reduce the tendency to store fat. You reduce your total fat and increase more metabolically active muscle tissue. The more muscle mass you build, the more calories you burn as a result of having more muscle mass, which burns more calories than fat. What wonderful compounding!

This even works when you're sleeping as it takes more energy to support your larger muscles. Approximately one-third of your day, when you are doing nothing except sleeping, your body is burning more calories. Now if we could just get back to earning six percent on our CDs.

MERLE'S STORY

Merle, now seventy-three, steadfastly refused to go to a gym. She would walk outside when the weather was good or on a treadmill in her home in the Boston area when it wasn't, but never in a gym.

Eight years ago she and her husband bought a winter home in SW Florida. She found that some days it was too hot to walk outside. Her husband reminded her that there was a beautiful fitness center down the street with lots of treadmills and she agreed to try it. She didn't have one at their winter home.

She learned that before she could utilize the facility she'd have to go through an interview process. The person who conducted the interview was Cathy, now the fitness director.

Cathy asked her if she would consider doing some strength training and Merle emphatically said, "NO!" Cathy then asked her a few questions: "Do you want to be able to pick up your grandchildren when they're toddlers? How about putting groceries in the trunk of your car?" Cathy got her attention and Merle added a half-hour of strength training to her half-hour treadmill work.

Merle had a bone density scan in her early sixties and was told she had osteopenia, a precursor to osteoporosis. It's less bone loss than osteoporosis, but still loss. She elected not to go on medication.

Two years after she started regular strength training she had another bone density scan and found that not only had the condition not gotten worse — the normal pattern — it had improved.

She started out using one- and two-pound weights and now does chest presses on a fitball with ten pounds. Not only has her strength improved but by incorporating an unstable surface during training, Merle's balance has improved as well.

THE FARMER'S DAUGHTER

If you own a farm you'd like to have some big, strapping sons for obvious reasons — field hands. Joan's father had not one but three farms and no sons but two daughters. I don't know how big Joan's sister is, but Joan checks in today at four feet, ten inches, 103 pounds. She said she was an able field hand anyway.

Joan can be a bit obsessive-compulsive — anything worth doing deserves 110 percent effort. She became a golf idiot (her words) at forty, a vegetarian at forty-six, took up aerobic and strength training in her early fifties. She sets goals for every physical activity every year, of course, that's what obsessive-compulsives do. She generally exceeds them.

Three years ago she discovered power lifting. For those of you who don't know, that means picking the heaviest weight you can lift for specific exercises: bench press, dead lift and squat. Competitive events require exact execution of each exercise.

This year Joan participated in an invitation-only power lifting event in Orlando and she walked away with a Bronze Medal in her class. She badly wanted to win but she did well.

Joan has long since given up being a golf addict. It now ranks after power lifting, general strength training and aerobics. Now seventy, she's in excellent physical condition, both fit and strong.

AN OCTOGENARIAN AND STRENGTH TRAINING

Sandy sent this story: "Some years back my then father-in-law, eighty-eight years old, a retired minister and artist, decided to build a display area on the road by his house for his sculptures. We cleared a space — probably eight feet by fifteen feet — and began building a stone wall to encompass it on three sides in order to present his works to the neighbors as they drove by. He worked several weeks on it with some local help — hauling stones to erect the wall about four feet high.

"One day toward the end he said to me, 'It's amazing, but I've not only developed muscles again, but I feel much stronger.' He never did a lick of serious exercise in his life, but with just a few short weeks of weight training at his advanced age, he got stronger. I was profoundly impressed and encouraged. As you say, it's never too late!"

WHAT'S A GOOD PROGRAM LOOK LIKE?

A spreadsheet summarizing a series of exercises for core, upper and lower body is included in the appendix. These are examples; books listed in the appendix will provide others as well as specific directions for doing them.

Some exercises, like seated row, require a machine. Others can be done with a machine, bar bell or dumbbells. Begin using machines for most exercises as it's easier to do. After a few months, consider using dumbbells where appropriate. Using free weights initiates more use of balance, important for proprioception.

Pick several exercises each for your core, upper body and lower body. Note what weights you use and track how many sets and reps you do. Set up a spreadsheet on your computer or graph paper to record the information.

Allow about an hour for warm-up, stretching, strength training and cool down. This includes core exercises, discussed in the next chapter. You need at least ten minutes in a light aerobic exercise like a treadmill or stationary bike, ten minutes for cool down stretching and about forty minutes for strength training and core exercises. That's a good workout.

The reason for having more exercises than you should do in one session is to provide variety for your brain and your body. It's more fun doing different exercises rather than the same thing every time. Take your time and do the exercises correctly. An hour out of your day is not a lot. Once you get used to it, the time will fly.

LET'S REVIEW

- Muscle loss begins in our forties and picks up speed every decade thereafter. That's why strength training needs to be an integral part of your exercise program — for the rest of your life.

- Balance and coordination are a big deal. Our bodies do it automatically via a process called proprioception. Aerobics and strength training help us maintain this ability as we age.

- There are two types of muscle fibers, slow-twitch and fast-twitch; we need both. Fast- twitch fibers tend to diminish more with age due to lack of use. Strength training is the best way to minimize the loss.

- Lifting weights to fatigue breaks down muscle cells so that they grow back stronger. It also helps in building stronger bones, ligaments and tendons.

- A trainer can be a big help with an exercise program. Getting started properly, staying motivated and doing exercises correctly is the best way to avoid injury. Using a trainer at least every two months to update your program is a wise investment. If you can't afford a trainer, get one or more of the books referenced at the end of this book and use it.

- Keeping records is a big deal and is easy to do. It keeps you honest with yourself, plus seeing improvement is motivating.

- The old axiom, "Use It or Lose It," applies to muscle and bone strength. You need physical activity in order to slow and even reverse the bone loss and muscle atrophy effects of aging.

ONLINE CLASSES

Physiic.com — $5 to $12 per class. Live classes in yoga, Pilates, strength training and aerobics.

Demandfitness.com — $15 per month. Classes in strength training, aerobics, martial arts and many more.

Yogalearningcenter.com — $8 per month. Video classes in yoga and Pilates.

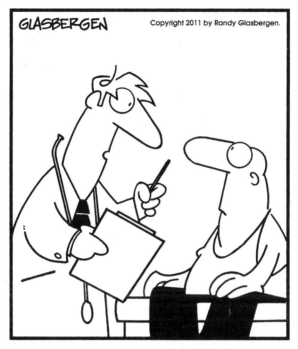

"Actually, golf is a great way to
exercise...if you use a bowling ball."

CHAPTER SEVEN — CORE EXERCISES AND OTHER GOODIES

"The first wealth is health." — *Ralph Waldo Emerson*

HERE'S WHAT'S COMING

- Let's be clear about what "core" means, and why it's so very important.

- How do you maintain balance as you age, a critical factor for independence?

- Should you do yoga?

- What's so big about stretching regularly, and how do you do it?

WHAT'S A CORE?

The core is the center of your body, from your shoulders to the bottom of your hips. Implementing a series of core exercises is right up there with strength training in importance. It's a great way to avoid back, shoulder and hip problems in your adult years.

Some of the issues addressed by core exercises are balance, stability, posture and abdominal strength. The lower back is a big one for all of us, maybe the most common area of complaint as we age. People who regularly do core exercises experience fewer physical problems and also increase their range of motion.

It's your core that's called on in almost every activity to transfer effort from one part of the body to another. This includes running, cycling, kayaking, golf and tennis. In golf, your core is what generates power for the hip turn that provides acceleration to your club. The power originates from the center or core. While the abdominal muscles are important, they are by no means acting alone. The core is all of the muscles that stabilize the spine and pelvis.

Core Performance by Mark Verstegen is a book that does a great job of outlining exercises for what he calls the "pillar" — the center of the body (the core) plus hips and shoulders — as well as for strength training overall. A trainer will definitely include core exercise as part of your routine. If you choose to develop your own, then Verstegen's book or a similar one will be very helpful.

Core exercises can be done at home while watching your favorite sport on TV. A fitball is a big help for this and is inexpensive to buy.

DISC PILLOWS, FITBALLS AND BOSU BALLS

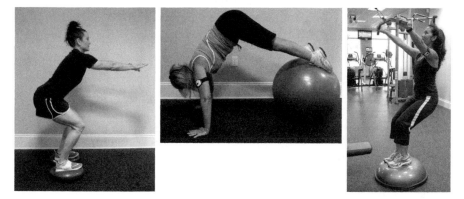

Disc pillows — They're circular, inflated and are designed to improve balance and coordination. Many exercisers stand on them while swinging a golf club, lifting free weights or using exercise bands. Don't be discouraged if at first they seem hard to use — keep working at it. Like most everything in exercise, frequency and persistence lead to improvement.

Fitball — Also called a physioball, it's a terrific exercise tool. Every gym has them in various sizes geared to the size of the individual. You can use one for lots of exercises, including but not limited to strength training and core exercises. For example, you can do bench presses and military presses lying or sitting on a fitball. The fitball requires balance during the exercise and, as a result, you use more muscles and nerve fibers in the process. This improves your proprioception, which we talked about in Chapter Seven. This is the ability to sense the position, location, orientation and movement of the body and its parts.

Bosu Ball — It's a half-moon, designed to be used both round side up and down. You can stand or sit on it for balance work while doing exercises or turn it upside down and do pushups from it. Every gym has them. Consider doing exercises like bench presses on this ball versus the fitball; you're closer to the ground if you lose your balance and fall.

Some of the most important muscles in your body are not involved with producing movement. They're critical because they provide the stabilizers we need for movement. The real benefit of using the equipment above is that you're forced to balance just like you are in everyday life, doing things like getting out of bed or standing on tiptoe to put a dish on the top shelf. One friend said that the balance exercises have reduced his fear of falling and he now feels more in control.

BALANCE FOR NONAGENARIANS — AND THE REST OF US

When Art's mother Martha was in her mid-nineties — still alert and very articulate — she got fitted for a hearing aid. At the same time they gave her a balance test and recommended a series of exercises to improve her balance. She did them regularly and her balance improved dramatically.

Some of the exercises involved using a bosu ball or fitball to sit or stand on while pulling on rubber cables. Others were standing on one leg with a cable attached to the other, then pulling in various directions. The balance muscles in the stable leg got stronger. A simple one but not so easy: stand on one leg and close your eyes. You won't last long initially but can dramatically improve your time, and balance, by doing it regularly.

Art decided to do them also and got the same result. He found a few more exercises, added them to the regimen and still does them. His stability in his kayak, a tricky little boat, has improved significantly.

The real benefits from balance exercises are in everyday life. It's easier to recover from a slip in a parking lot or a stumble on a set of stairs. It's also easier to stand on one foot and dry the other when getting out of the shower. You might even be able to walk across a creek on a log, like you did as a kid.

An orthopedist friend said that it's very difficult for older people to recover from a broken hip due to a fall. Balance exercises will help keep that fall from ever happening.

WII FIT FOR GRANDPARENTS

Ever see the Wii programs that run on your television? They have bowling, golf, baseball and many more. They also have a program, "Wii Fit." Gretchen Reynolds wrote a column about it, "Phys Ed: Why Wii Fit is Best for Grandparents." Reynolds reported that while Wii Fit was better for kids than sitting on a couch, there's not enough energy expenditure to keep children and teenagers fit.

An experiment involving eleven healthy elderly volunteers and fifteen undergraduate students, both groups fit, showed that the elderly subjects were in good shape but scored poorly on balance tests. When the two groups used Wii Fit for a few sessions the elderly ones improved dramatically, lowering their "Wii age" by eight years. The younger subjects only lowered theirs by one year. The age score was based primarily on balance tests. This would be a natural to do at home when you don't have time to go to a gym.

Ron added: "We purchased the Wii to have when our grandkids visit and for our own benefit.

"While the exercises contained within Wii Fit may not be an 'end all,' the basic components of what it sets forth are outstanding and mirror much of what you discuss in your book — Yoga, Strength Building, Aerobics, Balance.

"I've used the Wii Fit off and on for over a year. I think that if I could make myself stay with it there would be progress. The other good thing that it does is offer an easy way to keep track of what you're doing. The 'Body Test' feature measures your BMI and Weight and then provides graphs to trend your results.

"The Wii Fit also has 'beginner' and 'advanced' options as you work through the programs. I think many of your readers may have been exposed to the Wii as a result of their grandkids."

YOGA FOR THE OLDER GENERATION

Rich, fifty-eight, has been attending yoga classes for three years, three times a week. He was, and still is, normally the only male in the room. His story:

"Yoga is a breathing exercise that will make you more flexible plus will strengthen your spine and core. It will also improve your physique and improve your overall strength from the bottom of your feet (yes, your feet!) to the top of your neck. It will also help the mind and spirit. If you've been under stress for any reason, this is for you.

"A friend had told me how demanding yoga is, how much he perspired in a class (which I found hard to believe) and how revitalized he felt afterwards. I went to a class and was amazed at how difficult but enjoyable the yoga was. I walked out of my first class with my shirt soaked in sweat. Here are the types of yoga:

"Gentle Yoga — Yoga studios may have a very light workout called gentle yoga. There is very little exertion in a gentle class and may be good for someone who has never exercised and is in need of testing what they can handle.

"Hatha Yoga — This is traditional yoga. If you can walk a fifteen-minute mile you can handle a Hatha class. Hatha is demanding — someone who is very fit will get something out of it. Skip poses when you start to lose your breath, which you will. If you start to breathe too heavily slow down or stop; it's not a race. After you start breathing normally, jump back into the class.

"Vinyassa or Flow Yoga — At the studio that I attend these classes are demanding for seniors — not impossible but demanding. From a relative standpoint, if you consider yourself in the top twenty-five percentile of fitness for seniors, you can handle Vinyassa.

"Ashtanga Yoga — This is the highest level. It's very demanding, moves very quickly and all practitioners have a lot of experience. If you are in tip-top shape, are very flexible and have low body mass index, this may be for you when the Vinyassa is no longer a challenge.

"Yoga is NOT a competition or all about stretching.

"You'll struggle when starting out with yoga but don't be concerned if the person next to you looks better on the mat. They're glad you're there because when there are more in a class there's more energy.

"I was going to a chiropractor every six weeks but haven't gone in a year. Little aches and pains in my arthritic knees have gone away. If I drop something I can lean over to pick it up with no effort. Turning around in the car to look behind is easier with my range improvement of thirty percent. My upper body strength has increased fifty percent, my weight loss is five percent without eating less and my waist is two inches less and I sleep better.

"With regular yoga, you are slowing the aging process and improving your quality of life.

"We have a one-year-old grandson. As he was getting older and heavier my wife had a hard time holding him. She has started going to yoga with me about half the time and has built up strength so that our grandson is now easier to handle. She was very flexible to start so the strength improvement was the plus for her.

"I don't see many seniors in the classes, but I believe that anyone over fifty will really benefit from it. If you are intimidated by the process, go off to the side of the class. Just get there early to stake out where you want to be situated. For me, it's demanding so I go right to the front like the motivated kid who struggles in school and sits in front of the teacher to avoid distraction."

Rich didn't mention Bikram Yoga, the most popular form of hot yoga. Classes run ninety minutes and ideally are done in a room heated to 105 degrees Fahrenheit with forty percent humidity.

Maureen said:

"I'm glad that you included some yoga in your core chapter. Yoga is awesome for core strength and balance and also for your psyche. The yogis make it look easy but it is actually quite hard if done properly and you don't cheat. You should have seen Randy sweat in class!! He was fifty-eight at the time and there were four or five guys in the class. I have to get back to some classes — doing it at home is not the same. That probably holds true with most exercise. If you're in a group or a class you work harder.

STRETCHING

The benefits of consistently including stretching as part of your exercise program are considerable. Big ones are increased range of motion, reduced injuries, less muscle soreness and pain and fewer lower back problems. Others are improved appearance, body alignment and posture.

Ever have sciatica? It's generally caused by a compression of lumbar or sacral nerves. Common causes are a bulging disk, muscle spasms or lifestyle. Sitting on a big wallet may aggravate sciatica, or standing for long periods every day. Sciatica pain runs from the buttock on the side affected down the leg. One of the treatments is physical therapy and stretching exercises. Those who've had sciatica are generally highly motivated stretchers.

When you stretch the objective is to elongate the muscles and associated tendons. Initially the muscle resists, but if you hold the stretch for a period of time it will begin to relax and lengthen. Over time it will become easier to lengthen that muscle, but remember, it takes time. Trying too hard can lead to injury.

Proper breathing is an important part of the process. Muscle fibers need oxygen to be stretched and they get it by you breathing deeply during the process. Muscle fibers lengthen when they're stretched, but some fibers remain at rest. The more the fibers are stretched, the longer and more useful they will become. This happens over time by repeated stretching.

Elizabeth added: "You could mention the importance of keeping your eyes open for balance, breathing slowly and deeply to allow the body to lengthen on its own. Don't force the stretch. You'd be surprised where your hands/fingers end up from where they began at the beginning of the stretch. Slowly come up, using your core so you don't injure your back."

A good trainer will likely recommend stretching before and after a workout. It's also easy to work some stretching exercises into your workout. Be sure you've warmed up for at least ten minutes prior to doing any stretching. At minimum, make ten minutes or more of stretching a consistent part of your routine at the end of a workout. There are several types of stretching:

Static stretching — This is the traditional method many of us have used. Let's say you bend over to touch — or try to touch — your toes. Hold that stretch for a few seconds or longer and then straighten up and do it several more times. Many books and trainers recommend holding a stretch for fifteen to thirty seconds.

Dynamic stretching — This is done while performing sports-specific movements. An example would be swinging two golf clubs in order to warm up the back and shoulders prior to playing. Dynamic stretching is essentially the same as performing a warm-up for a sport but at a lower level of intensity.

Active-isolated stretching — The object is to contract the muscle that is the opposite the muscle to be stretched. The isolated muscle will relax. Stretch it gently and quickly, holding the stretch for no more than two seconds, and then do it again. An example is contracting your quadriceps while stretching your hamstring.

Which is best? Static stretching is generally preferred because there's less chance of injury and muscle soreness. Many of us perform dynamic stretching regularly when we warm up for golf, tennis, cycling, etc. Research studies have shown that thirty minutes of static stretching exercises performed at least twice a week will improve flexibility within a very short time.

It's very helpful to have a book with illustrations to guide you through stretches. A number of them provide sports-specific illustrations and directions. I'll include a list at the end of this book.

THE IDEAL WORKOUT

There is no one ideal workout but there are elements of one. *First, a strong aerobic workout — ideally including some anaerobic time doing intervals — should not be done on the same day as strength training.*

A vigorous aerobic workout leaves your body tired and that's not an ideal time to take on yet another hard workout, particularly if you've graduated to doing strength training to fatigue. That doesn't mean that a warm-up for strength training shouldn't include time in an aerobic activity — treadmill, stationary bike, arc trainer, etc. But the purpose is to get your blood flowing and raise the temperature of your muscles in order to lessen the chance of injury.

Aerobics — What's your exercise of choice? If you're working indoors in a gym you have lots of options. The key is to find something you enjoy. Ideally, find several and vary them so that your body doesn't get too comfortable. A good aerobic workout should involve at least thirty minutes at an aerobic and anaerobic level. This means about ten minutes to warm up and reach a minimum of sixty percent of your maximum heart rate and then a few minutes to cool down at the end, allowing your heart rate to drop below sixty percent of MHR. A total of forty-five minutes is a good workout.

If you're working outdoors — running, cycling or brisk walking — you may spend considerably more time exercising than in the gym. Being outdoors is conducive to that, provided the weather cooperates. Many of us do outdoor aerobic activity when weather permits and indoor activity when it doesn't. Few of us would enjoy riding a stationary bike or walking on a treadmill for two hours, but we might well spend that much time exercising outdoors on a beautiful day. In either case, allocate ten minutes or more for stretching at the end.

Strength training — Including your warm-up, core exercises and stretching, this should range from forty- five minutes to an hour.

After some warm-up exercises, do some core and balance exercises and then strength training. By that time your muscles are nice and warm and you'll reduce the potential for injuring a muscle during strength work. Then finish with some stretching to cool down.

LET'S REVIEW

- Core exercises are a mandatory part of any strength training program; that's the center, from your shoulders to the bottom of your hips. Good conditioning of this section of the body is critical for every transfer effort; running, cycling, kayaking, golf and tennis.

- Yoga has significant benefits for flexibility and strength. If you have access to classes, consider giving yoga a try.

- Stretching during and after a workout should be done every time.

CHAPTER EIGHT — SUPPORT GROUPS AND CONNECTIONS

"Here is the basic rule for winning success. Let's mark it in the mind and remember it. The rule is: Success depends on the support of other people. The only hurdle between you and what you want to be is in the support of other people."

— *David Joseph Schwartz, Ph.D., author of* The Magic of Thinking Big

HERE'S WHAT'S COMING

- A support group can make the difference between thinking and doing.
- There's a formula for success with a support group.
- Learn about a new concept — The Village Movement.
- Staying connected with friends and family is a big factor in staying healthy, mentally and physically.

A LIFETIME OF SUPPORT

You may not have thought of it this way, but we've been in one big support group all of our lives. Most of us have had family, friends in school at all levels, sports coaches, co-workers who served, formally or informally, as coaches or mentors and, of course, our spouses. Much of what we've achieved in life can be traced directly to the support of others. Dr. Phil said recently, "Set your life up and surround yourself with people who support you." While many individuals achieve success in fitness and healthy eating going solo, there's no question that the odds of success increase with involvement of one or more partners.

PLAY TOGETHER, STAY TOGETHER

Kathy said, "Do you think there's an opportunity to write for men and women in a way that would appeal to couples exercising together?

"I realize that the over-fifty set begins to do a lot of things separately, but it would be great to provide a perspective on how friends, partners or married couples can motivate each other to stay on track. As you know, research shows that cohabitants usually weigh similarly due to common eating and exercise habits . . . it's hard to change one without the other.

"Jeff and I have literally walked hundreds, if not thousands, of miles together since we got our first pair of Labrador Retrievers in 1992. We're now on our second pair and we still walk them miles every day and longer on the weekends. We go to the gym separately due to work schedules, but exercising together (walking, biking, golf, whatever) is great time spent with your partner. Just an idea . . . from someone who's still romantic!"

A recent *New York Times* article reported that full-service gyms are now losing more members than they can replace with new ones. About forty-five percent of gym members quit in any given year and fewer than that are signing up. One consultant places the heart of the blame on the fact that everyone's now plugged in, either to their IPod or the flat-screen television located on their exercise equipment. Less socializing means less support, which leads to lower attendance; eventually many drop out.

Lots of research has shown that we do better when we're involved in a support group. Some examples:

- A total of forty-three companies implemented one of two smoking cessation programs. One involved participants viewing a television program and using a self-help manual. The other used these materials plus had six self-help group meetings. The twenty-one companies who used the group meetings had a forty-one percent rate of smoking cessation versus twenty-one percent for those who used a television program and a self-help manual. Three months later an average of twenty-two percent of the meeting group participants had continued not to smoke versus twelve percent for the others.

- An informal analysis of Alcoholics Anonymous has shown that the more participants attend AA self-help meetings the longer their sobriety. Those who take an active role and also provide support for others do even better.

UNFAMILIAR TERRITORY

If you walked up to a ten-year-old and asked if they would like to do something they'd never done before, the automatic response would be, "Sure!" from most of them. Young people like to do new things but as we age the rules change. We become more careful and cautious, less inclined to do things we've never experienced before.

Exercise can be a good example of this. Going to a gym when you've never done it before can be very intimidating. It seems like everyone except you knows what they're doing.

Taking up a sport like cycling or running can be equally intimidating. New cyclists have understandable concerns about riding in traffic or falling and suffering an injury. New runners think about potential damage to their joints. Walking is the only physical activity where the number of participants increases as we age.

Art added: "Our gym has a very large contingent of seniors who don't know a lot about what they're doing, but they arrive en masse, take a class, learn and have the support of their group. They laugh at themselves and others in good spirit."

RICK'S SUPPORT GROUP

Several years ago Rick, in his mid-sixties, took stock and decided he'd get in shape. He revised his eating habits, started going to a fitness center regularly and in a few months he dropped thirty pounds. He's kept the weight off since then.

Rick had done a bit of cycling but had never gotten serious about it. He knew that I was an avid rider so he approached me one day and asked if I would ride with him, which I was happy to do. We did a few short rides at a moderate pace to get him acclimated.

Rick went to a bike store and bought the works: a high-end carbon fiber bike and all of the accoutrements. He got a good helmet, shoes with clip-in pedals, shorts, jerseys and gloves. He knew that if he purchased a really nice bike it would motivate him to stick with the program, and he was right.

Rick started riding several days a week with our group. He struggled to keep up initially but we'd wait for him and give him a chance to catch his breath. Within a few months he was able to do a sixty-mile ride, way beyond anything he would have imagined. A bit over a year later he did a century — a one-hundred-mile ride.

Would Rick have been able to do this on his own? Not a chance. Having a group to encourage him made all the difference.

ELEVEN/ELEVEN AND FIFTY BY FIFTY

Sally decided on November 11, 2007, that she was going to lose fifty pounds before she turned fifty years of age on October 15, 2008. She had eleven months to do it. The weight had built up slowly over a thirty-year span of having kids and not exercising.

She told her friend Janice who said, "I'll do it, too!" Her support group was formed. She picked a winner, a friend who cared about her as well as herself.

Sally decided she wanted to be fit more than fat. She visualized how she wanted to feel and what she wanted to look like. She then just told herself to go — don't think about it, just go. At least six days a week she got out of bed, put on her shoes and hopped on her treadmill. Every other day she also did strength training.

The other big step was building the muscles in her two hands — to push away from the table so that she didn't eat too much. She cut down on the quantity plus eliminated food like potato chips and ice cream. They were still in the house for her teenage kids but she pretended they weren't there. If there was a birthday cake for someone at her office she drank the coffee and skipped the cake.

She missed her goal; on her fiftieth birthday she'd lost forty-five pounds. But when she thought about it, she'd added at least five pounds of muscle by doing strength training, so she'd really lost fifty pounds or more of fat.

Sally and Janice decided they should do something new, so they signed up for a year of thirty minutes three times a week at Curves. The next year they joined the LA Fitness gym near work where they go three times a week for aerobics and strength training. Like everyone Sally has had some lapses, but she and Janice always get each other back on track. Having someone who cares makes a huge difference.

A FORMULA FOR SUCCESS

Here are some ideas for moving into unfamiliar territory:

- Look for friends who are doing what you'd like to do. Ask for their help; most will be glad to provide it. In fact, one-hundred percent of your real friends will.

- Take up an activity with your spouse. Bill H, an avid tennis player, golfer and fitness participant, initiated a daily walk of two to three miles with his wife to help her become more fit. Bill Y and Halyna motivate each other to go to the fitness center regularly.

- Look for an established group. Many communities have cycling and runners clubs for all levels of ability, for example. Use Google to check these out.

- If you're considering joining a fitness center, call them and ask if someone will show you around. Use one of the most powerful sentences in the English language: "I need your help."

- If you can't find an active group in the exercise area you want, start one. Think about who you know who would benefit from doing what you want to do.

CINDI ON RUNNING

Here's an inspiring story from Cindi, a woman in her forties and a resident of a New York suburb, who started a running support group for women in her town: "Running has been a huge part of my life as long as I can remember. I've completed ten marathons and many other races.

"Over the past few years many people have asked me running-related questions and always seem fascinated with my long runs and training.

Many of them have said to me, 'I wish I could run,' 'I always wanted to run a marathon,' 'I'm not a runner,' etc. As I crossed the finish line of my last marathon a light bulb went off in my head. I needed to somehow share with others the joy that running has brought to my life.

"This year I decided to start a running program in my town. I've joined running groups in the past and loved training with others. I enjoyed learning about other people's lives as well as learning about myself during the process.

"My running group started as a simple idea and has grown very quickly. We now have eighteen members; we meet twice a week. Once a week we do speed work and hills and on those days I incorporate things like yoga, stretching and nutrition. Then on the other day we do our 'long' run.

"The long run is different for everyone. I go out running before we meet. I take chalk and mark off every one-quarter mile up to eight to ten miles. This way they don't have to think about how far they are going — it is there for them and if they want to go just a little farther each time they can bump it up a bit and then turn around.

"Then the group meets, everyone talks and decides who wants to run what and they break up into groups and run. I've been sticking back with one person who runs slower and is very new to running. I don't want her to get discouraged so I stay with her. As the club progresses I will map out longer runs.

"Watching how these women have embraced the confidence that they've gained from running with this group is amazing. The pride and accomplishment they gain from showing up and pushing themselves further than they ever imagined has impacted them in other aspects of their lives. The group is so much more than just about running. It's about camaraderie, goal setting, building confidence and learning that, with a little support, you can accomplish anything.

"My goal was to be the middle person between whatever was stopping them from setting these goals and reaching them. When you accomplish physical things you thought were impossible, it gives you the confidence to accomplish other things in your life. That's what I want to give to these women. Everyone in my group will run a race by the end of the program so they feel what it feels like to cross their own finish line."

LAUREN'S STORY

This is Lauren's story of what Cindi did to get her hooked on running:

"When I say that I really never ran before joining Cindi's running group, I am not stretching the truth. I really did not run. I mostly did the elliptical, tennis, spin class, body fit and other non-running activities. I would sometimes walk around the neighborhood.

"When Cindi approached me about her running group, I told her that I'd never run. She said that anyone could run. I was skeptical. I really didn't think that I could run around the block, let alone a mile or more. She told me to just give it a try. I wanted to show support for my friend's new endeavor, so I gave it a shot.

"It certainly hasn't been easy. I'm definitely the slowest person in the group, but with Cindi's inspiration, I've run four miles. I also ran my first 5K and I did it in a great time for me! She always says that anything is possible and I believe it. The other women in the group are great. When we run around the high school track and they run past me they are always so supportive. My next goal will be a 10K and I really think that as Cindi says, 'anything is possible!'"

PAUL'S TWO CENTS ON SUPPORT GROUPS

Paul is a resident of the San Francisco Bay area. A former priest and a recovering alcoholic, he's been a terrific contributor to this book. Here's his story about support groups.

"I didn't discover support groups until I was forty-five. Over the past twenty-five years they have been a huge part of my life. Support groups have raised my self-esteem and have taught me that everyone has problems.

"I've often wondered if I was in the bathroom when the teacher handed out 'rules for living.' Support groups now give me new rules for living. If I'm going through a new experience I can usually find someone else in the group who's already had a similar experience and can adapt that person's experience to the new situation in my life.

"The support groups that I like tend to be non-judgmental and free of editorializing. I tend to choose those groups that contain people who emphasize experience over ideas or lecturing. I like my groups to be void of 'shoulds' and be groups that, though occasionally confrontational, are light on criticism of others in the group.

"I also tend to choose support groups that will give me unconditional friendship and those where there's no money attached. Nobody is obligated to do anything for anybody else, and participation in the groups that I attend is free and for fun.

"After I attend a meeting of one of my support groups, the feeling that I have when I walk out is: 'Boy, I'm glad I don't have the problems those people have.' I've heard it said that in a good support group, if you asked everybody to list their problems on a piece of paper and to place their paper in a pile in the center of the group, and then asked everyone to choose which problems they'd like to have, everyone would likely take their own problems back."

PAUL'S SUPPORT GROUP FOR ALCOHOLISM

"I've been able to stop all drinking completely since my very first meeting. Before that I drank alcohol every night. I've learned how to be a better husband in my marriage of over forty years.

"Shortly before entering this support group my marriage was in shambles and in danger of being dissolved. I've learned to be a better father to my two children. Prior to my entrance into recovery my relationship with them was strained. At the time of my diagnosis, my eleven-year-old son said to me, 'Dad, I didn't know you were an alcoholic; I just thought you were a jerk.'

"I've also learned how to be a productive worker at my job. Nearly seven years into my recovery, I received an award from the president of my company for being the best sales rep in a company of 300+ reps. Prior to my attending meetings, my job security was in great jeopardy due to my drinking. About fifteen years into recovery I found an ex-boss (who happens to be the author of this book) and was able to make amends for my inadequate work on the job some twenty-five years before. Today I consider Harry one of my best friends.

"These successes happened because I've sat in rooms listening to other alcoholics pour out their problems and give their experiences of what life was like when they first came into these meetings and what they've been able to do for themselves by sitting in these meetings. I listened to people in their very first meeting and learned how horrible their lives are. When a newcomer speaks for the first time, you can hear a pin drop. That's because everyone in the room is busy comparing themselves on their first day to the experience of that newcomer.

"I love the saying 'People who don't go to meetings aren't around to hear what happens to people who don't go to meetings.'

"I have no idea what most of these people do for a living. I don't even know the last names of most of them and I usually don't know where they live. I don't know if they're rich or poor or what kind of cars they drive or how much their houses cost. Yet when I run into them at the airline ticket counter, at Safeway or at the gas station I know all about them.

"Eight years ago I was in the hospital after a heart attack. The stream of visitors to my room was steady — day and night. The front desk attendant came to my room to ask if I knew the people that she was sending to me. A lot of people were asking to see 'Paul,' but nobody could tell her what Paul's last name was."

Another friend, a woman, added this after reading Paul's story:

"A friend took me to a support group that she believed was helping her stay away from alcohol. It quickly appealed to me also. Remember the Verizon ad on television that showed an infinite number of supportive people standing behind the caller in the network? Anytime I romanticize the notion that a drink might be a good idea, I envision that network (support group) behind me encouraging me to stay the course. Having a support group has had a dramatic impact on the quality of my life."

INTERNATIONAL SUPPORT

Ruth said: "Currently, my own improvement program includes the positive reinforcement of a buddy. We speak on the phone briefly every weekday to say, 'I did it!' She lives in Canada and has free long distance with no international charge. We understand it's just as easy and better to develop a good habit as practice a bad one. My friend has totally worked up a regular yoga program for herself; in my case, I'm working on daily walking and stretching in addition to my twenty minutes a day of personal writing. Just knowing the 'I did it' call is coming is an amazing motivator. And we never lie.

"Ron and I have been healthy eaters for many years now. He had a near-fatal heart attack sixteen years ago when he was fifty-seven. Both of us are low fat, low salt, highly vegetarian diners . . . with a glass of wine now and then. Protecting ourselves against 'slide' is our most difficult task, so motivational reading is valuable. I tell you this so you know where I'm at in my own personal thinking and awareness. Brushes with death will do that for one."

CHANGE OR DIE

This is the title of a book by Alan Deutschman. The subtitle is *The Three Keys to Change at Work and in Life.*

Deutschman presents compelling evidence as to why fear is not a strong long-term motivator for many people to change, even in the face of death. An example would be someone who suffered a near-fatal heart attack, survived, and now has a chance to modify his or her behavior by implementing exercise and healthy eating. Fear may motivate them short-term, but many simply can't handle the fear because it's too overwhelming. They tend to revert to their former habits, no matter the outcome. There are certainly exceptions to this as evidenced by several stories in this book. The problem is that they are the exception versus the rule.

Deutschman tells the story of how Dean Ornish, a professor of medicine at the University of California San Francisco, has had excellent results using a team of experts to provide support: a fitness trainer, a yoga teacher, a chef or nutritionist, a psychologist and a group of patients with similar problems who work to help each other. Ornish sells them on the "joy of living" versus the "fear of dying."

When we think of support groups we often think of Alcoholics Anonymous, which has been providing support for those with alcohol and drug abuse problems for many decades. While they don't publicize the results of their interventions, they likely are one of the most successful ways of dealing with these issues.

The key steps outlined by Deutschman are:

Relate — Form a relationship with a group who can provide the support and encouragement needed to implement change.

Repeat — Implement the new behavior until it becomes a habit. The Alcoholics Anonymous slogan for this is "Fake it until you make it." Remember that a habit is simply a behavioral autopilot.

Reframe — Ornish talks about the "joy of living." He works with patients to get them to understand how much better their life can be if they are healthy. He's a terrific salesman, among other things.

All of us are not in a position where we fear death due to a debilitating illness, nor are we able to marshal a team of experts to lead us down the path of exercise and healthy eating. But what I learned from this book was the enormous benefit we can obtain by becoming involved with a group of individuals with similar issues and concerns — a support group.

WHAT'S MOST IMPORTANT?

We started a program at our fitness center in SW Florida this spring called "Living a Healthy Life." The goal of the program is to provide an opportunity for members to change and enhance the quality of their life.

We began with an assessment of the current fitness of the thirteen participants: height, weight, blood pressure, flexibility, recovery time from aerobic activity, etc. We then had an introduction to a software program where each person can record their daily food and liquid intake. We've had seminars by doctors, nutritionists and fitness specialists, special fitness classes for the participants, individual fitness coaching from a personal trainer as well as group meetings to discuss progress.

At the end of eight weeks we had an assessment to measure progress. The results were terrific in every category: weight lost, body fat reduction, increased strength and endurance. Every participant elected to continue in the program. We'll provide support each month with activities similar to those in the first eight weeks.

New programs have been started each month for a dozen participants and the fall programs, which is the time when many return to SW Florida, are oversubscribed. The buzz in the community is that this is really good. There's now a waiting list for the fall programs.

What have the participants enjoyed the most, and mentioned most frequently, that they want to continue? The support group meetings.

REINVENTING CAROLINE

Here's what one participant, Caroline, had to say about the program: "A new pilot program, 'Living a Healthy Life,' was started at our local fitness center and I was asked to be one of the participants. My initial response was that I didn't think I could do it and I turned them down.

"I'd been athletic most of my life, playing competitive tennis for the past twenty years as well as golf, skiing and biking; I had prided myself on my abilities and fitness. However, recurring injuries and a serious chronic back issue had severely limited my ability to participate and I reluctantly stopped all sports at age seventy.

"I figured I would keep in shape by going to the gym. Yes, I was getting a bit of a muffin top, but doesn't that come with age anyway? I was also getting more and more bent over with my deteriorating back. I assumed this was just the price to pay for age and sports injuries. I had a minimal program I followed at the gym and felt that was all I could possibly do.

"I was strongly encouraged to join the program in spite of my health issues and, as a result, my life has turned around. A personal trainer developed a program that compensated for my disabilities and the support of a group of similar ages encouraged me to exercise beyond what I thought I could do, in a safe environment.

"I now stand up straight — for the first time in years — have a strong core that supports my back and a much higher level of overall fitness. My muffin top is almost gone!

"Of course, I still have my chronic back problem and arthritis, but I just FEEL better — stronger, happier, have more energy — a real change from just giving up at seventy and feeling that's just the way it is. With the help of a well-designed program and the support of a group with similar goals I've been reinvented!"

Six months later Caroline added: "It's hard to believe that it's now six months since I started the program. I've lost twenty pounds, now have sculpted arms and, most important, a very strong core that allows me to stand up straight in spite of degenerative disc diseases.

"To my surprise it's been quite easy to continue with healthy eating and exercise. Once the results started to be apparent, I couldn't wait to get to the gym and keep going. Group members continue seeing each other at the gym, complimenting and supporting our progress and success."

BECOMING A GYM RAT

Diane, another participant in 'Living a Healthy Life,' said: "I've worked hard, been diligent and the LHL program has produced results. I feel better, am healthier and have more energy. My clothes fit better and my husband is very complimentary.

"I love the new friendships I've developed with the others in the program. We have fun laughing together about successes and frustrations. I've been so proud of what others in the group have accomplished and hope that I was a part of their success. We cheered each other on and became a team.

"Circuit training was fun and an out-of-breath experience. It was a great chance to reconnect with everyone in the program. I remember watching as one of our group crawled from station to station, making us all laugh. We had FUN!

"The day someone — you know who you are — said that I'd become a gym rat was one of my proudest moments! Me? Yes, me! Fitness has become a part of my life."

Working with others changed Diane's life — the power of a support group.

STAND TALL

Bill H, Diane's husband, added: "My goals were to get fit, change my exercise protocol, increase the intensity, prepare for a biking trip to France and lose weight. I have taken steps forward to meet each of those goals.

"In addition, I learned a lot about my poor eating habits and how important nutrition and changed eating habits are to success. I make much better choices in foods, portion sizes and learned when not to eat as a result of listening to others and the experts involved in the LHL program.

"My posture has improved, I feel taller and my clothes fit much better. I put on slacks that I haven't worn for twenty-five years and wore those out-of-date madras to a costume party, much to the delight and ridicule of my friends. My agility and speed on the tennis court has improved to the point that my frequent playing partners recognize my ability to reach balls which had previously been out of reach. In biking, I am back to being able to do interval training in a standing position on the few hills in SW Florida.

"It's a wonderful program conducted by an energetic and interested staff in a superb facility. I'm excited to interest others in this behavioral and life-altering experience."

THE VILLAGE MOVEMENT

A new concept for seniors was started in Beacon Hill Village in Boston in February 2002. A group of volunteers organized into specialty areas like help with home care, technology, transportation, walking dogs and many others. Each participant pays a membership fee; rates for paid services are negotiated and are standard for all members. There are now over fifty Villages organized around the United States. Example cities are Berkeley, Palo Alto, San Francisco, San Diego, Washington, Denver and Coral Gables. The goal is to provide the services needed for seniors to stay in their homes and live independently longer.

While the primary focus of the movement is on providing seniors with the ability to live independently via economical services, participants also benefit from the social companionship involved.

If you'd like to know more about how to start such a program in your community, go to the Beacon Hill Village website. You can order a Founder's Manual as well as a Supplement to the Founder's Manual.

STAYING CONNECTED

Social connections play a big role in staying healthy, physically and mentally. Studies have shown that those with less social contact are more prone to mental illness. A big factor in depression problems is a lack of social interaction, particularly with family. Other studies have shown that the higher the level of social interaction, the higher the cognitive performance.

SAPOLSKY ON SOCIAL CONNECTIONS

A friend referred me to a very interesting and well-written book, *Why Zebras Don't Get Ulcers: The Acclaimed Guide to Stress, Stress-Related Diseases and Coping* by Robert Sapolsky. He's a professor of biology and neurology at Stanford and a former recipient of a MacArthur Foundation "genius" grant. He's also a research associate at the Institute of Primate Research, National Museum of Kenya.

Sapolsky's book is loaded with interesting information. Among them:

- Fewer social relationships lead to a shorter life expectancy as well as worst outcomes as a result of infectious diseases.

- The results of limited social relationships are comparable to major factors such as smoking, obesity, hypertension and a low level of physical activity.

- The immune response system of those who are socially isolated is much lower. Studies have shown this with antibody response to vaccine, people with AIDS and women with breast cancer.

- The size of social networks is smaller with age but the quality of the relationships tends to improve.

- The average level of happiness tends to increase with age. Older people have fewer negative emotions and those they do have tend to not last as long.

DON'T WAIT

Mike was raised by kind and loving parents. He always knew he was adopted but really had no interest in contacting his birth parents. He figured they had rejected him, so why bother.

Then two events took place in a short time period; his adoptive parents died and he turned fifty. He decided he would like to know more about where he came from and knew he had better do it sooner than later. His natural parents, if they were still alive, weren't getting any younger.

He contacted Social Services and learned that the terms of the adoption specified that any contact with his birth mother was her decision, not his.

He also learned that his natural father had died and that he had deserted his mother when she became pregnant out of wedlock.

After several months of encouragement his mother called him but was reluctant to meet. He learned that she had not told her husband or two children that he existed. It was no surprise that she was reluctant. He also sensed that she had been carrying a big load of guilt over having given him up.

When she confirmed the guilt he said, "Phyllis, you have no reason to feel guilty. You did the right thing under the circumstances." Mike said he could almost feel the relief on the other end of the phone; fifty years of guilt melting away.

After Phyllis had time to inform her husband and children they had a family reunion — Mike, his mother and his half-brother and half-sister. Mike said they treated him like a member of the family immediately.

Several years ago Mike had decided to get in shape. He lost fifty pounds and now cycles over 8,000 miles per year. His half-brother Jim is heavy, like Mike used to be. Mike offered to help by providing encouragement and education. Jim is now into cycling and is making progress on his weight.

Mike said, "On my new 'new' family: I speak with my siblings several times a week and usually chat with Phyllis at least once a week. It's magical. They've welcomed me and my family with open arms."

FIFTY YEARS OF CONNECTIONS

Art passed on this story about his wife Sue: "Almost fifty years ago my wife Sue was accepted late at Gettysburg College, her first choice college. When she arrived on campus the dorms were full. The college had purchased three houses very close to campus and housed about thirty females who had all been accepted late. Sue joined eight others in "West Cottage," a small house that had beds and desks for eight freshmen girls, two bathrooms and a resident advisor.

"These nine girls lived together for just one year back in the early 1960s. A funny side note is that four of them were named Susan. All were quickly given nicknames to keep things clear and today, almost fifty years later, they still call each other by those names.

"Seven of the nine stay connected with get-togethers organized almost every year, plus have phone calls and email updates the rest of the time. Husbands have bonded with other husbands and are invited to attend the official college reunions held every five years. These girls are clearly the power group when attending reunions at the Gettysburg campus — a group thrown together by circumstance remaining close friends for fifty years."

STAYING CONNECTED — INTERNET STYLE

While many of us have utilized email as a way of staying connected with friends and family for some years now, more sophisticated connections have become enormously popular in less than ten years.

Facebook, founded in 2004, has become the most popular social network website in the world. They now boast over 135 million unique monthly visitors; over forty-two percent of the U.S. population has a Facebook account.

MySpace, launched in 2003, initially was the most popular social website but was superseded by Facebook in 2008, based on monthly unique visitors. MySpace is estimated to have about 43 million unique visitors monthly.

Twitter, launched in 2006, offers social networking and microblogging service, allowing users to send and receive messages called "tweets." These are text-based, up to 140 characters. Twitter is estimated to have 190 million users worldwide who generate sixty-five million tweets daily.

YouTube, launched in 2005, allows users to upload, share and view videos. In order to upload videos you must be a registered user, but anyone can view them.

LinkedIn, launched in 2003, is primarily for professional networking. LinkedIn has over 90 million registered users and boasts over twenty-one million unique visitors in the United States and forty-eight million in the world.

A survey of reviewers of my manuscript leads me to the view that these social networking sites are less popular with older adults. Many say they don't want to take the time and don't see the value. A few — not many — make very little use of technology.

Remember the Curve of Pistophenes in an earlier chapter? This is the frustration of learning something new and getting "pissed off" as we go through the process. Some say, "Why bother? I've got enough social connections in person and through emails."

One reason to bother is that it may prove the most effective way to keep in touch with the younger friends and family. Think grandkids; they jump on new ideas and technology like a fish to water.

A FACEBOOK STORY

Art said the following about utilizing Facebook: "I use Facebook to reconnect and stay connected with a group of friends, mainly bike riders/racers, from the years that I was active in the sport and industry. Also in the mix are friends from high school, college and earlier careers. It's certainly a less personal connection than I have with my closest friends, but a number of Facebook connections have led to closer personal relationships.

"A few months ago when we were casting around for a realtor to help sell our property in New Jersey, I asked a Facebook friend who still lived in the neighborhood for a recommendation. She provided one and he worked out very well — the property was sold. Somewhere in the process we began a regular correspondence and I learned that she and her significant other spend the month of March near us in Sarasota. Last night they came for dinner. We hadn't seen each other for fifty years. It was like we never missed a beat and just took up where we left off. Ken, my best friend since kindergarten and who has since passed away, was Jane's sweetheart in high school. We shared lots of old Ken stories."

SOCIAL CONNECTIONS AND WEIGHT

A study of young adults eighteen to twenty-five found that those who were overweight tended to have overweight romantic partners as well as overweight best friends. This trend even carried to their casual friends and family members.

Those who were overweight were more motivated to lose weight if they had social contacts who were also interested in losing weight. Would this hold true for adults? I suspect that it would. Weight Watchers made a large business out of this.

SOCIAL CONNECTIONS AND PAIN

A study at UCLA was done with twenty-five women, mostly UCLA students, who had boyfriends with whom they'd been in a relationship with for at least six months. They received a moderately painful stimulus on their forearms while they went through a variety of conditions. In one they viewed a picture of their boyfriend, a chair and a stranger. In another they held their boyfriend's hand, the hand of a stranger or a squeeze ball.

The results were that the women reported less pain when they were looking at a picture of their boyfriend or holding his hand. So, if your partner can't make it when you go to the doctor and expect to experience pain, take along a photo.

BILL COSBY

Shortly after graduating from Temple University in 1993, my son Michael was working in the New York area in television production. He met Bill Cosby and worked on his short-lived TV show, "You Bet Your Life," a remake of the original show done by Groucho Marx years ago. Cosby was very nice to Michael; he had him to his home several times in the Philadelphia area.

Once, when Cosby was meeting with a senior producer at his house and Michael was sitting off to the side, not wanting to be in the way, Cosby said, "What are you doing sitting way over there? No, no, you come here and sit next to me; you're here to learn."

Cosby is also a graduate of Temple University. Michael now resides in San Francisco and was co-president of the Temple Alumni Group for four years. The group attended a Cosby performance in Oakland and Cosby gave them a private reception prior to his comedy show. It was a perfect opportunity for Michael to thank him for his hospitality, friendship and for helping him learn, his real contribution.

Michael said, "One thing you might add to the Cosby story is the willingness to give back. I did by becoming President of the Northern California Alumni Association in order to get the 1,800 Temple alumni in the Bay Area reconnected to Temple. That's what led to seeing Cosby eighteen years later at his comedy event."

THE COUNSELOR

My son Michael came to live with me and my second wife Deb when he turned fourteen. At the time we were living in Annapolis, MD, a terrific place. We had a sailboat on the Chesapeake and were in the process of building a home in a waterfront community.

He was just beginning his sophomore year in high school. I said, "Michael, whatever happens, we'll stay here until you finish high school," a dumb statement if there ever was one. Soon after saying that I was offered a career-changing opportunity in Naperville, IL, and we moved at the end of his sophomore year.

Michael had ADHD and some other learning disabilities that made school a challenge for him. High school was tough; he was fortunate to have Bill, a terrific counselor. Bill, Michael and I met a number of times to discuss suitable colleges for Michael, and he ended up attending one Bill recommended. When that didn't work out as planned Bill helped him think through his next options.

Over twenty years later Michael tracked down Bill and met with him to thank him for what he'd done for him. He learned that Bill, then eighty-five, meets his replacement every Thursday at 5:30 AM for breakfast to find out how things are going.

Michael said this about staying connected: "I'm not sure I have a great story, other than just that I'm involved in people's lives. I'm genuinely interested in them and what they are doing. Facebook is a huge help on this, but that's different.

"I've found staying in touch to be a thread throughout your life and mine long before Facebook. Sometimes I know I have relationships that are a one-way street but I accept that and realize I enjoy them and accept my role as the initiator."

In the July/August 2009 issue of *Scientific American*, an article reported that "Individuals who are optimistic, agreeable, open to new experiences, conscientious, positively motivated and goal-directed are more likely to undergo successful aging, to take advantage of opportunities, to cope more effectively with life circumstances, to effectively regulate emotional reaction to events and to maintain a sense of well-being and life satisfaction in the face of challenge."

These same individuals are the ones who will reach out to maintain connections to current and former friends, do volunteer work and maintain an active role in their community.

JUST SHOW UP

Bill Y has lived in Madison, WI for many decades. Over thirty years ago he was invited to join a support group that was initiated as a result of the involvement of some men he knew in the Young Life program. They'd become active with their children and consequently formed close friendships with each other.

Bill's now a resident of SW Florida but still participates with the group when he's in Madison. When he or others are unable to personally attend the meeting, they often will do so via a teleconference. The core group of five has been together since the beginning, with the exception of one who died recently.

Others have joined over the years but many have not been comfortable sharing their thoughts. The group never has an agenda, except to talk about whatever is on their minds. They know that all information they share is confidential within the group, so they feel safe discussing a range of topics.

Bill added: "Over the years we've dealt with a wide range of issues ranging from death, terminal illness, mental illness, addiction, loss of jobs, business losses, divorce and many other issues common to our everyday lives. Each of the five have experienced one or more of these issues and benefited greatly from sharing with the others.

"The keys to the success and longevity of the group are: 1) mutual respect; 2) confidentiality; 3) shared experiences together; 4) belief in

God; and 5) a commitment to simply show up.

"Being involved with a group of men committed to being there for each other has been a blessing for all of us. Each of us has experienced loss which has been made more bearable by being able to talk about our feelings with others who listen and offer support. Attending as often as we can is high on our priority list.

"As I think about the group, the real key to our group's longevity is the commitment to show up. Many times we had schedule conflicts, but the group succeeded due to the desire of each person to make the weekly meetings a priority. The same applies, it seems to me, to living a healthy lifestyle . . . just show up."

SOCIAL CONNECTIONS AND HEALTH

Researchers at the University of Chicago reported that those who feel lonely face bigger health problems. But those who are able to adjust to being alone don't have the same issues.

The most socially connected are three times as likely to report very good or excellent health compared to those least connected. This applies also to those who've adjusted to being alone. The study involved about 3,000 people between fifty-seven and eighty-five years of age.

Even blood pressure is impacted. The university researchers reported that even those with a modest level of loneliness had higher blood pressure than those who were most socially connected.

RELIGION AS CONNECTION

Several studies have shown that the friendships built in a religious setting provide satisfaction. Those who have several close friends in their church express a higher level of satisfaction than those who don't.

Henry has been a neighbor in SW Florida for eight years. We live in a community renowned for its golf activity and a high percentage of the residents are very active in the sport, but Henry isn't one of them as he doesn't play the game. This has placed limitations on his social involvement with individuals in the community. Many eat, sleep and dream about golf.

His wife Alice suggested that they get involved in a local church and Henry agreed, primarily because Alice wanted to do it. He'd not been an active member of a church for many years. Henry soon found that he thoroughly enjoyed the church and has become a very active member. He enjoys participating in weeknight dinners and has helped with a number of the church's fund-raising activities.

The reason is primarily the connections he's made with several members. They've become close friends; they're connected.

LIVING FOR SOFTBALL

The *Naples Daily News* had a recent story about "Earl the Pearl." Earl, ninety-one years old, has been playing softball for over eighty years. He said, "Softball means everything. If I didn't have softball I'd be dead by now."

Earl has been part of many championship teams over the years, including an over-eighties team in Fort Myers, FL, in 2001 and 2003, that won the Eighty-Plus World Series Softball Tournament in Iowa.

Today he doesn't run the bases anymore but has a substitute after the first base. He plays right field versus left as there's less activity. But he plays and enjoys the friendship and camaraderie of his teammates. It's his most important social connection.

LET'S REVIEW

- You can significantly increase your chances of succeeding at starting — and staying — with an exercise and healthy eating program by finding others to join you.

- Maintaining social connections is not only important for your mental health. People with strong social connections are much healthier physically also.

- The internet is here to stay. If you haven't already, consider testing one of the social networking sites as a way of keeping in touch with others, particularly the young.

- *Scientific American* got it right: "Individuals who are optimistic, agreeable, open to new experiences, conscientious, positively motivated and goal-directed are more likely to undergo successful aging."

CHAPTER NINE — OVERCOMING LIMITATIONS

"It's not what you accomplish in life but also what you overcome."
— Johnny Miller, TV announcer and former professional golfer

HERE'S WHAT'S COMING

- Let's define "limitations."

- If you currently don't have any limitations, should you read this chapter?

- What does "The Butterfly Effect" have to do with exercise?

- We'll cover a variety of health problems and give inspirational examples of how individuals are overcoming their limitations and leading an active, healthy life.

WHAT'S A LIMITATION?

We'll define a limitation as a condition that keeps an individual from doing something he or she would like to do, or maybe from doing something in the same way as those who don't have their particular condition.

The conditions we'll discuss include hypertension, hypotension, arthritis, heart disease, osteoporosis, osteopenia, Type I or Type II diabetes, back problems, strokes and Parkinson's. You may ask; "Harry, I don't have any of these problems, so why should I read this chapter?" Good question.

The answer is that it's likely that you or members of your family will have one or more of these problems during your lifetime. Many of them can be avoided by taking proper action now — exercising properly and eating healthy. We can be sure that no matter how carefully we tend to our physical state, we will all at some point encounter a condition that presents us with a limitation.

Chris, one of my cycling friends, said, "Most of us have to deal with a health problem at some point and many of us with multiple ones. The key is to not let them get us down. "There's no magic pill for many of the diseases and conditions that follow, but exercise and healthy eating come close. Virtually every health issue discussed in this chapter benefits from exercise, both aerobic and strength training. Some can be prevented by combining these with healthy eating.

A doctor's advice is required prior to implementing a significant exercise program. Frequently it's not a matter of whether but when. Those recovering from a stroke or heart attack, for example, need coaching on what to do and how much.

Research studies show that at least one-third of us will have Type 2 diabetes. One source said that ninety percent of us will have high blood pressure at some point in our life. Reading about problems others have had, many likely more severe than any we'll experience, can provide sound knowledge and meaningful insight as well as inspiration.

These are among the most powerful stories in this book. I was overwhelmed by the passion and enthusiasm these individuals have for what they're doing to maintain an active lifestyle. Exercise has clearly changed their lives. They're a model of what we all can and should do.

THE BUTTERFLY EFFECT

Many have heard the metaphor about a butterfly flapping its wings in South America and becoming the beginning of a hurricane days later in North America. Weather is difficult to predict for long periods in advance because of the difficulty in measuring the starting atmospheric conditions accurately. This has to do with extreme sensitivity to initial conditions.

We know that small differences in an early health-related condition can produce large variations later on. The butterfly effect is a good way of thinking about your exercise, diet and other health habits that you form today. They'll have a big impact on your future and you want to manage these initial conditions as much as you can. There are no guarantees, but it's better than leaving it to chance.

Let's say you're currently sixty years of age and enjoy reasonably good health. We'll assume you do some exercise and think about what you eat but aren't religious about either issue. Your blood pressure is a bit high but you're not on medication and you could stand to lose twenty pounds. Let's also assume you enjoy wine and a few snacks before dinner. You normally have two glasses of wine before dinner, along with some cashew nuts, and one glass with dinner.

The three glasses of wine total about 360 calories; an ounce of cashews is 150 calories, 110 of which are fat calories. Three ounces of cashews is a small serving, but let's use that total. This means that the wine and cashews total about 800 calories. The wine is primarily carbohydrates while the nuts are primarily fat. That's 800 out of a total of about 2,500 calories per day as a normal intake.

What would happen if you reduced the wine to two glasses and eliminated the cashews or just had an ounce of them? You could substitute carrot sticks or butterless popcorn as a snack. This would reduce your daily calorie intake by about 400 calories, or 2,800 per week. In a month, conservatively, that would add up to over three pounds.

What if you simultaneously decided to make exercise a regular part of your life by walking two miles every day? That's about 200 calories per day or 1,400 per week. In a month that would be close to two pounds of fat burned. Think about it — that's sixty pounds in a year reduction in wine and cashews plus the exercise. It's likely that your body would adjust to your lower intake during the year and reduce this total somewhat, but it would still be a significant number.

While these may be small changes today, think about the impact they would have on your health years from now. **Your new, leaner body will be much less prone to most of the health problems we'll discuss in this chapter.**

HOW DID I SURVIVE?

Cathy is the director of our fitness center in SW Florida. In 2004, she was in a serious auto accident that could have been fatal. She credits her fitness from her exercise program for her survival. Here's what she said:

"After seeing pictures of what was left of the car...how did I survive? I always weight trained heavy and did plenty of cardio...my trapezius muscles were very strong and kept my neck from snapping . . . another great reason to work out . . . even if you're a girl! (The trapezius is a large muscle that spans the neck, shoulder and back.)

"After my accident I could no longer teach classes since I couldn't remember sequences and patterns for a routine, a major part of instructing aerobics classes. By participating in group classes and working with qualified personal trainers I continued to improve my memory . . . being told to grapevine right, walk forward eight, tap four, walk back four, grapevine left and step up right . . . my neurotransmitters were firing like crazy — my brain was telling my extremities to perform the correct patterns.

"I couldn't complete these patterns with the speed or consistency as before but I was at least experiencing improvement and my love of exercise (sweating, even if girls aren't supposed to), getting my heart pumping and oxygen to my brain and muscles — exercise is brainpower."

Today Cathy is fully recovered, mentally and physically. She continues to work out regularly and encourages others to do the same. Exercise before the accident contributed significantly to her survival; exercise after the accident allowed her to recover and live a full life today.

NO BRACES, NO CANES

I'm sure somewhere there's someone who's had more health problems than Bob, but I've never met him or her. Bob, now seventy, has had hyperthyroidism, ulcers, chronic kidney disease and a heart attack that required two stents. That's just for openers; three years ago he was diagnosed on Christmas Eve with a very aggressive form of prostate cancer for which he had radiation treatments. That same year he contracted Type 2 diabetes.

Two years ago he had a detached vertebra, followed by a spinal rupture that required surgery. The latest was drop foot, a form of neuropathy. He was told that he would have to wear leg braces and use two canes for the rest of his life.

Bob, who'd never had time for exercise, decided two and a half years ago that he was going to make time for it. He met with a trainer at our fitness center in SW Florida and started a serious exercise program. He goes to the gym here or in Massachusetts three or four times a week and does an hour of serious strength training and stretching. He does three sets of ten reps each of a series of exercises using heavy weights. He also does exercises at home on the other days.

Bob said, "The combination of strength training and stretching has dramatically changed my ability to lead a full life, including playing golf. I've made some swing adjustments due to my back but otherwise I play the same as always."

Bob said that it helps him to use a trainer every time he goes to the gym. It's his way of being sure he shows up; he has an appointment. What about the braces and canes? Contrary to the prediction of two doctors, he has no need for them.

I wondered whether the exercise had also improved his blood glucose levels. Bob said: "As you might expect, I respond to challenges with gusto. Blood glucose levels are measured by an 'A1C' test. An A1C value of 6.5 or greater is used for the diagnosis of diabetes. When I was diagnosed, my A1C value was 12.1. That diagnosis was another impetus to begin my exercise regimen and it also brought about a major change in dietary habits. Three months later my A1C was 5.7; my endocrinologist said that he had never seen that sharp a drop in so short a time. It's never risen as high as 6.5 since."

In terms of motivation, exercise has moved from extrinsic — something he does because it's good for him — to intrinsic — something he does because he enjoys it. Having witnessed what exercise did for her husband, Bob's wife Janet has joined the team and she now goes to the gym regularly as well.

HYPERTENSION

Frequently called high blood pressure, about one in three adults in the United States have it. It's sometimes called the "silent killer" as there are no symptoms. Some people feel a tingling in their extremities — that's a warning sign. The problem is more prevalent as we age. Men and women over forty-five are more likely to develop it and women over fifty-four are more likely to have it than men. Data from the Framingham Heart Study shows that even if your blood pressure is normal at age fifty-five you still have a ninety percent chance of developing hypertension during your lifetime.

Major factors contributing to high blood pressure are family history, ethnicity, obesity, diet, stress and inactivity. We can't do anything about family history or ethnicity — African Americans have a higher incidence than other ethnic groups — but we can do plenty about obesity, diet, stress and inactivity.

Blood pressure is an indication of how hard your heart is working as well as the condition of your arteries. It's a simple formula: C x A = B. Cardiac output times arterial resistance equals blood pressure. Each beat of your heart pumps about five ounces of blood into your arteries; that's about four to five quarts per minute of normal activity. If you're involved in strenuous activity your heart pumps a lot more in order to meet the demand for oxygen.

Arterial resistance is the pressure the walls of the arteries exert on the blood. The less flexible your arteries are, the greater the resistance and the higher the blood pressure. If your arteries are narrow or inflexible it will be indicated by your blood pressure numbers.

There are two measurements in your blood pressure. Systolic, the higher number, is when the heart contracts and pumps the blood into the arteries. Diastolic, the lower number, is when the heart is refilling between contractions (beats).

DO THE NUMBERS:

- Normal — Under 120/under 80
- Pre-hypertension — 120–139 / 80–90
- Stage 1 – 140–159 / 90–99
- Stage 2 – 160+ / 100+

If your blood pressure is at stage 1 or stage 2, it's time to schedule an appointment with your doctor. He or she will likely recommend diet and lifestyle changes as well as perhaps a medication to bring it down.

Blood pressure tends to rise with age, but exercise and healthy eating can reduce the chances of this happening to you. Some of us have what's called the "white coat syndrome." The tension of being in a doctor's office leads us to produce higher numbers than normal. I'm one of those people. That's why I have a blood pressure monitor at home so that I can periodically check my numbers. You can obtain one for under $100 in a pharmacy.

Blood pressure is lower following vigorous exercise and the difference can be significant. My normal is in the low 120s to low 70s but is in the mid-110s to the mid-60s after a two-hour bike ride. If you don't choose to purchase a monitor you can take your blood pressure for free at most pharmacies, many grocery stores, as well as some gyms.

Many of my cycling friends in Florida and Pennsylvania have hypertension, likely due to a family history as most of them are in good to excellent condition. They take a medication to control it but most, with their doctor's approval, take it after their exercise. Blood pressure medications slow down the heart, reducing blood flow, not what you want when you're exercising hard and need blood flowing to your muscles. All of them have checked with their doctor to be sure delaying the medication is okay.

Diet and Obesity — These two are under our control. A diet issue that has reappeared recently in the health and fitness news is the role of too much salt in our diet. Salt tends to cause our body to retain water. The excess water within and surrounding our cells puts pressure on our blood vessels and this pressure increases resistance to blood flow and can contribute to hypertension.

Many can reduce their blood pressure by significantly reducing their intake of salt and by eating a diet high in fruits and vegetables. Obesity contributes to hypertension because the enlarged fat cells also put pressure on the circulatory system, increasing resistance to blood flow.

Regular exercise is very beneficial in reducing hypertension. A reduction in body fat is an outcome of regular exercise. Every time a skeletal muscle contracts it assists blood flow by the "milking action" on blood vessels. Skeletal muscle activity squeezes the blood in the vessel, propelling it along. When the muscle relaxes, the blood refills the blood vessel; another muscle contraction and the refilled blood in the vessel is propelled forward.

All of this contributes to enhanced blood flow and decreased heart muscle strain to propel the blood. With regular exercise your heart gets stronger because you're challenging it. Your blood flow is enhanced and your hypertension is reduced.

Stress — One of the best antidotes for stress is exercise, both aerobic and strength training. That's true, of course, for about everything in our life. Those of us who've been in high-stress jobs at one time or another and have maintained a regular exercise program know how powerful regular exercise can be in managing stress. Exercise can also help us maintain perspective when we have disagreements with family members.

HYPOTENSION

Much less prevalent but worth mentioning is hypotension or low blood pressure. A reading of ninety or less for systolic pressure or sixty or less for diastolic is considered hypotension. Recommendations are to drink lots of water and limit consumption of alcohol, a diuretic, eat a healthy, low-carbohydrate diet and increase your salt intake. While fruits and vegetables are carbohydrates, they also have lots of water. Aerobic exercise is also recommended.

CORONARY HEART DISEASE

This may be new information to you as it was to me: *heart disease kills more people each year than all other causes of death combined, including all cancers.* Lifestyle plays a huge role in this disease, which is the single most preventable cause of fatalities. The keys to avoid this one, no surprise, are exercise and healthy eating.

Some of the most active exercisers I know have had coronary stents installed or had coronary artery bypass surgery. Aerobic and strength training exercises are now a recommended component of the recovery process for coronary artery disease. Other approaches to recover from or prevent coronary heart disease are diet changes and medication. Counseling helps, providing insight as to the how and why of lifestyle changes.

"Tim's Great Awakening," whose story is in Chapter Two, was particularly inspiring. Tim was fortunate that his ninety-eight percent blockage in two arteries was discovered in time. He's now the picture of health, having dropped thirty-five pounds and implemented — with his doctor's blessing — a serious aerobic and strength-training program.

INTERVALS AND HEART PROBLEMS

Some of you are likely thinking, "Harry, every time I turn a page you're talking about intervals again; enough already." Sorry, but here we go again.

A June 28, 2011, article in the *Wall Street Journal* by Katherine Hobson titled "To Heal a Heart, Train Harder," talks at length about the power of short intervals in improving the fitness of heart patients.

The big advantage of intervals for those of us who have a healthy heart is that they improve both our speed and endurance. It turns out that the same is true for many who've had heart problems. They improve their ability to transport and utilize oxygen efficiently, a big deal. Several studies have shown that those who utilize thirty-second, high-intensity intervals periodically during their exercise improve their use of oxygen more than those utilizing a moderate-intensity program. The number of intervals and their length are gradually increased over time.

A patient at the Mayo Clinic in Rochester, MN, who'd had double-bypass heart surgery, showed dramatic improvement doing one minute of high intensity every five minutes of aerobic exercise. In about seven weeks of exercise following his surgery, his resting heart rate went from eighty-four beats per minute to fifty, his average heart rate during exercise went from 120 to 107, the number of intervals from none to five, and the total time of exercise from twenty minutes to thirty-five minutes.

This technique has been utilized with proper supervision by the Mayo Clinic for four years, but a number of other locations and doctors are not yet convinced. Be sure you discuss this with your cardiologist before implementing any change to your program.

THE POWER OF TOBACCO

Gary, seventy-four, has had more than his share of health issues; kidney disease, forty years of back problems, plus a blockage of an artery to the heart that doesn't lend itself to successful surgery.

He quit his habit of smoking three packs of cigarettes a day in 1977, but replaced it with chewing tobacco for twenty years, then replaced that with five cigars a day. He finally quit all tobacco in 2006. He acknowledges that tobacco likely contributed to a number of his health problems. "After I had surgery in 1997, to open a ninety-nine percent blocked carotid artery, I began being concerned about all of the tobacco and the rest of my system, but with no symptoms, I and my doctors assumed all was OK."

His back problems were improved by a series of steroid injections, but his heart and kidney issues required him to take on a personal commitment to more intense physical and dietary action. In January 2009, he got serious about exercising and healthy eating. He dropped thirty pounds in four months and has kept them off.

Gary now swims a mile three times a week in a respectable fifty-three minutes, plus he walks three and a half miles three times a week in slightly over an hour. His doctors are delighted with the improvements in his cardiovascular system as well as his kidney functions. According to Gary, "My back and my golf swing have been fortunate beneficiaries of the exercises and aerobics."

His heart knows it needs more blood flow and, as a result of his aerobic exercise, has grown supplemental collateral arteries from other areas of the heart to at least partially compensate for the blocked one. With the less-than-positive "risk/reward" results of any open heart surgery, in his case, Gary is very upbeat when he smiles and says, "I really enjoy and appreciate my new lifestyle, especially when I realize that if I continue it, I can die with my heart condition instead of from it."

OSTEOARTHRITIS

The medical profession doesn't understand what causes osteoarthritis — the loss of cartilage around joints — nor is there an effective treatment. The hard shiny cartilage on the bone ends at the joint is somehow eaten away, leaving raw bone ends. This isn't very encouraging news if you have the problem. About twenty-seven million adults in the United States have the problem, which leads to 632,000 surgical joint replacements annually.

Historically the recommendation was that those with osteoarthritis "take it easy," but the new mantra is "get moving." An article by Laura Landro in the *Wall Street Journal* on April 12, 2011, provides an excellent summary.

As Landro reports from Kate Lorig, director of the Patient Education Research Center at Stanford University: "The most dangerous exercise you can do when you have arthritis is none." Losing weight is also a big deal as each extra pound of weight adds the equivalent of four pounds to the knees. Studies show that women are at higher risk of knee problems than men.

Strengthening leg muscles via a strength-training program has proven beneficial for those with arthritic knees. Stronger muscles stabilize the knee, reducing movement at the joint and increasing function. Swimming and cycling are good choices as they're not weight-bearing exercises. Walking is good also, as long as it's not painful. Set a moderate pace at the beginning of any of these and take a break if you need it. A slow, steady approach produces the best long-term results.

Many communities have self-management programs and others are available online. These provide information and classes as to which exercise programs may be best for you and which should be avoided. Self-management programs have a very positive effect — they've improved the health of patients by fifteen percent to thirty percent over the use of medication only.

Tai chi — This is a Chinese form of meditation therapy that involves slow, rhythmic movements and stretches designed to build strength and flexibility. Classes may be available at your gym, senior center or YMCA. Research has shown this to be helpful in reducing pain and stiffness as well as in improving balance. It's a complex exercise that also aids brain fitness.

Yoga can aid in stretching the hamstrings, as well as knees, shoulders, neck and back. Stretching can be a big help in relieving discomfort after exercise.

Art added: "We took a Tai chi course while we were in the Peace Corps in Suriname and it was perfect. In one sense it was a stressful time, learning a new language and adapting to a new culture. We got stronger, more relaxed and I've never slept better."

STEVE'S CYCLING CAREER

Steve was a very strong cyclist, the strongest sprinter in our group in SW Florida. Sprinters are the guys who can go fast for a short distance. He'd leave us in the dust.

Then some health issues arose, as they have a tendency to do. He had surgery for prostate cancer followed shortly after with surgery for a hernia. Osteoarthritis in an ankle got worse, making it difficult for him to walk any distance. He said, "It's bone on bone." His exercise program went south as his weight moved north. Not surprisingly, he lost motivation.

The good news is that it's not as painful for him to cycle as it is to walk. A few months ago he started showing up regularly for our rides. His endurance was not what it used to be, naturally, but he kept at it. He can't leave us in the dust as he used to when sprinting but he's back trying.

One of our cyclists is seven years his senior (that would be me!). Steve's motivated by the fact that he can't out-sprint me the way he used to. He said recently, "Harry, you wait; when I lose ten more pounds, you're toast!" He's already dropped twenty pounds and plans to lose twenty more. I'm delighted to be a factor in his motivation and look forward to the day he can dust me again. Well, maybe "look forward" is a bit of an overstatement.

Steve added: "Harry, the only time my ankle doesn't hurt is when I'm chasing you up that overpass. The adrenalin flow is so great that I can't feel a thing."

Steve's condition was so severe that he recently elected to have an ankle replacement, a relatively rare surgery. As of this writing he's recovering well and expects to be back cycling in a few months.

PARKINSON'S

One of the best treatments for Parkinson's is an exercise program involving both aerobics and strength training. Stronger muscles improve the ability to move and can counter some of the effects that Parkinson's has on movement.

EXERCISE TRUMPS PARKINSON'S

Stu, sixty-six, was diagnosed with Parkinson's disease thirteen years ago. The progression was so slow, however, that they weren't positive of the diagnosis until six years ago.

Stu retired and started a serious exercise program shortly after a bout with pneumonia five years ago. He does three days a week of strength training and stretching, utilizing the services of one of the trainers at our fitness center in SW Florida. Five feet, five inches tall, he's moving weights that amaze those who watch him. He does short sessions of aerobics using the treadmill on the days he does strength work.

Stu also does three days a week of serious aerobic exercise. He's on the treadmill for fifty minutes, moving at over four miles an hour at an elevation of two to four degrees. His goal is to really get his heart pumping.

Stu has a massage once a week; massage helps to eliminate muscle stiffness and rigidity caused by Parkinson's. Massage also has a positive effect on the nervous system by helping to increase circulation. Stu said, "Exercise has canceled the progression of my disease. I'm as healthy today as I was five years ago and, of course, in much better physical condition."

Remember the earlier story about Sergey Brin, the co-founder of Google, and what he's doing to avoid contracting Parkinson's? It's in Chapter Four.

OSTEOPOROSIS AND OSTEOPENIA

One of the problems we can develop as we age is lack of bone strength due to the loss of bone mass. This is called osteoporosis or osteopenia in its milder form. It can be a big problem for elderly people as the likelihood of a fracture increases. It's easy to get tested for this problem. A friend said he had it done at a drugstore for about $30.

Two areas of the body are particularly susceptible: the spine and the hips. Compression of the spine resulting from bone loss can put pressure on the nerves exiting the spinal column. This in turn can cause chronic pain and muscle weakness. A hip fracture is a common occurrence following a fall and many who fracture a hip never recover; some remain bedridden and others never fully regain their mobility. In both instances independent living becomes compromised.

While a calcium supplement can be helpful, the best medicine is our old friend, exercise. The exercise needs to be weight-bearing, which is why strength training is so important. Weight-bearing exercise positively stresses the bones of the body, including those in the hips and vertebral column. In response to the good stress during weight bearing, the bones adapt and get stronger.

Couple this with good dietary sources of calcium, such as dairy products and dark green vegetables, plus a calcium supplement of 1,000 to 1,500 mg per day and you can reduce the risk and consequences of osteoporosis. An adequate supply of vitamin D is also essential for good bone health. Aging and the use of sunscreen limit the input we can receive from sunlight, a major source of vitamin D. Consider a supplement of 400 IU per day.

The sooner dietary changes and a good weight-bearing exercise program are started, the better. It's never too late to begin.

SWIMMING

Swimming is obviously not a weight-bearing exercise and, as a result, has not been viewed as helpful in increasing bone density. However, a study at the Veterans Administration Medical Center in Portland, OR, showed that males forty to eighty-five years of age who'd been swimming regularly for at least three years had significantly greater bone mineral density than did non-exercisers.

Dr. Susan A. Bloomfield is a Professor in the Department of Health and Kinesiology at Texas A & M University. In addition to being a Masters swimmer she does extensive research on bone issues. She said: "We have the current emphasis on either weight-training or weight-bearing activities that involve impact forces to provide adequate stimulus to the skeleton. A diversified exercise program that uses a wide variety of muscle groups with frequent and varied movement patterns would be better than a monotonous signal to bone like running or cycling."

TERRY'S OSTEOPENIA

Terry is in his fifties and is an avid cyclist. He fell on a mountain bike trail in California last year and had to be taken out of a canyon via helicopter. He learned that he had a mild hip fracture due in part to his having osteopenia. While he was in superb condition aerobically, he'd not done any strength training. Cycling didn't provide the weight-bearing exercise that he needed. He's rectifying that problem, of course.

If you currently have either osteoporosis or osteopenia and don't do strength training exercises, begin slowly. Hire a trainer who can get you started properly at an appropriate level of resistance. In addition to strength training, stair climbing, walking and dancing are good. They involve aerobic activity as well as being weight bearing. If you have access to yoga classes, give them a try.

BACK PROBLEMS

Probably no limitation is more prevalent among adults than back problems. Over eighty percent of us are likely to experience back problems at some point in our life. This can be the result of nerve, muscle, disc problems or arthritis. Lots of pain medications are sold to those with back issues.

A big problem is a herniated disc, a condition in which the outer fibrous ring of an intervertebral disc develops a tear, allowing the softer central portion of the disc to bulge outward. This bulge can lead to pressure on the nerves exiting the spinal cord. One of the most common of these conditions is sciatica. The result is pain in one side of the buttocks and down the leg. As someone who's experienced this condition I can attest that it's very painful. While the success of back surgeries has improved significantly in recent years, many of us are able to avoid that fate via exercise and healthy eating.

Probably the best exercise for those with back problems is swimming, which puts no pressure on any point in the back. Swimming laps builds up shoulder and back muscles, leading to better trunk support. Healthy eating is a big deal. Reducing any excess fat in the stomach is very important as the added weight pulls the body forward and strains the back.

Roger, an exercise kinesiologist, recommends strengthening the abdominal muscles as this produces a better alignment of the vertebra, particularly in the lower back, and takes pressure off the posterior side of the intervertebral disks, the likely location of herniation.

Roger added, "As uncomfortable as they are, some type of sit-up exercise or abdominal crunch exercise is necessary. The critically important part, however, is doing these with the hips in some degree of flexion. This position does two things: it makes the abdominal muscles work harder, which is good, and it reduces the forward pulling pressure produced by the deep hip flexor muscles, the iliopsoas muscle group. An example of hip flexion is to lie on your back and bend your knees toward your chest. In the process of flexing your knees you're also flexing your hip."

Many of the exercises done when lifting weights or on resistance machines are also good because you tighten the abdominal muscles to stabilize your trunk and, by doing so, you strengthen these muscles.

Ever wonder why very pregnant women will stand and put their hands on the back of their pelvis and push forward? They're straightening their lower back, the same thing good abdominal muscle strength does. Ever wonder why it feels so good, if you have a "potbelly" to lie on your back on the floor and just let your vertebral column straighten out? It's the same thing: backward pressure reduction on the intervertebral disks.

Weak abdominal muscles producing bad posture adds up over the years and greatly increases the risk of back problems later in life. It's never too late to start, but if you have a back problem, start slowly.

If you have extra body fat stored in your abdomen, exercise and diet will start to reduce it. The body fat in your stomach causes the lower back to curve forward, a condition called lordosis, and this puts pressure on the back of the intervertebral disk.

A cycling friend with a herniated disc was told by his orthopedist not to ride his bike. When he explained to the doctor that he experienced no pain either during or after cycling, the doctor changed his view. Cycling, if it isn't painful, has the advantage of offering excellent aerobic exercise without applying pressure to the injury.

David, an M.D., added:

"Harry, I've had a herniated disk in my lower back for fifteen years and there are two exercises that I like to do that cause absolutely no back pain — walking and cycling. I'm sure swimming would be great as well but I don't enjoy it."

STAND UP STRAIGHT

The New York Times published an article by Lesley Alderman, "Sit Up Straight. Your Back Thanks You" on June 24, 2011. Following are some of the key points.

While we definitely incur some back problems due to aging, most of the problems are because we've not developed core strength and good posture. These two go hand in hand. If we implement a strong core exercise program — think having a trainer provide guidance, or review core exercises in one of the books listed at the end of this one —good posture will follow.

An excellent suggestion is to avoid sitting or driving for long periods of time; take a break. If you're at home, get up, stretch and move around every thirty to sixty minutes versus sitting at your desk for hours. If you're driving, think good health versus setting a speed record.

My wife and I drive from Pennsylvania to Florida several times a year. We've worked out a plan where we stop at a rest stop every two hours or sooner and walk around. We've ditched the former habit of seeing if we can beat our "best" time. No surprise, we feel better at the end of the day. Our dog also likes the break.

A PERSONAL STORY

We've all had some level of back pain at one time or another, but when I was in my late forties mine moved from occasionally uncomfortable to frequently painful. An MRI showed that I had a herniated disc. The physical therapy my doctor recommended was terrific — like a deep-tissue massage — but the pain didn't go away. In short order I moved from over-the-counter pain pills to a full-fledged narcotic three times a day.

A surgeon almost had me convinced to undergo an operation but I got lucky. A doctor friend referred me to one of the top back guys in Chicago, where we lived at the time. After the most thorough examination I've ever had for any condition, he said, "This is heresy for a surgeon, but if I were you I would not have surgery. When we go in we create scar tissue, which may rub against the nerves in the same way as your bulging disc. You may be no better off."

He recommended three steroid shots injected into the herniated disc spread over three months. He also recommended swimming laps, which I initiated with a vengeance; pain can be a strong motivator. Within a short time I was swimming a mile three or four times a week.

The steroid shots were very helpful but the swimming was the life changer. Within a few months my pain went from an eight on a one-to-ten scale to a two and I eliminated the pain pills. Over a period of several years it got even better and I found that I could participate in sports like golf and cycling with no pain. My back and shoulder muscles had strengthened to the point that I didn't put strain on the affected area. If you have consistent back pain, try swimming. It might be the key to your living a full life.

ANN'S BACK

Ann read my story and added: "Eight and a half years ago I was facing spinal fusion because of severe sciatic pain and protruding discs. The neurosurgeon I consulted for a second opinion was pretty much like the one you mentioned in your book — too many people suffer just as much afterwards from scar tissue, collapsing discs further up the spine, etc. She strongly urged me to start lifting weights so I joined our local YMCA the very next day. About a year later, while I was working out, I heard a voice I recognized; I looked over and there was the doctor herself lifting weights."

ARTIFICIAL JOINTS

I wasn't surprised to learn that a hospital near my winter home in SW Florida performs the second-highest number of joint replacement surgeries in the United States. Knees and hips are the most common, although I have several friends who've had one or both shoulders done.

A number of the replacements are likely due to a high level of athletic activity in younger years. One friend ran what he described as "way too many" marathons and had to have a hip replacement recently. Another, a college football player, has had replacements for one knee and both shoulders.

Another big factor, no surprise, is body weight. Those who are overweight or obese are placing considerably more stress on their joints. A high percentage of the replacements are for adults in one of these categories. An extra pound of weight puts four pounds of additional pressure on joints.

RUSTY'S KNEE

The old axiom, "The harder you work, the quicker you recover" is spot on for knee replacement. Rusty, sixty-eight, showed up to cycle with our group recently only three months after a knee replacement. Here's what Rusty said:

"Before surgery I couldn't cycle so I swam about five miles a week. I also continued with strength training and Pilates, both supervised. After surgery I started physical therapy the next day. I continued after leaving the hospital with physical therapy three times a week as well as home exercises. My biggest issue was flexing; the extension seemed to be easier, so I could walk with a cane the second week after surgery.

"I was able to walk without assistance the fourth week. I believe the type of surgery helped some of the recovery. Biomet furnished my implant and my surgeon used a relatively new procedure called MRI Mapping. They map your leg from the hip to the ankle and the surgeon makes some notations and then it is sent to Denmark for complete measurements, which take six weeks.

"With this procedure no guesswork is needed by the surgeon; all of the dimensions and cuts are pre-done and the joint is specifically made for you. My surgeon had done forty of these and all were successful. Surgery was completed in less than forty-five minutes. It's been a relatively pain-free recovery but it's also been hard work.

"In contrast my sister Jane, seven years older, is overweight and out of shape. She had a knee replacement two years ago, then fell and broke her hip. She's never recovered and is in a wheelchair. Her good leg has atrophied to the point it will not support her and she's given up on physical therapy. It's very sad."

Remember the story "Tom — The Artificial Man" in Chapter Seven? He's overcome potential problems that could result from a hip replacement and two artificial shoulders by continuing a strong aerobic and strength-training regimen. The stronger muscles he's developed as a result allow him to lead a full life.

TYPE 1 AND TYPE 2 DIABETES

Type 1 Diabetes, also known as juvenile diabetes, early-onset diabetes or insulin-dependent diabetes, is a condition where the pancreas produces little or no insulin. It comes on quite suddenly, affecting children of only a few months old up through early adulthood.

Insulin is required in order for glucose (sugar) to exit the blood and enter cells for use as an energy source, or to be used or stored. Without insulin the glucose remains in the blood and diabetes is the resulting condition.

Type 1 diabetes is thought to be a result of both genetic and environmental factors. The Beta cells of the pancreas, which produce insulin, are damaged, often by a virus, and permanently destroyed by the immune system. This results in a lack of insulin.

Individuals with Type 1 diabetes must supplement the shortfall of insulin via daily injections or the use of a pump that regulates their input of insulin. There is no cure for Type 1 diabetes, but individuals who take care of themselves can lead an active and healthy life.

Type 2 Diabetes is a condition where the individual's body doesn't respond properly to the effects of insulin. Type 2 diabetes has been called adult-onset diabetes and non-insulin dependent diabetes. In this condition there is resistance to insulin and glucose doesn't enter cells but remains in the blood.

A Type 1 diabetic will have high blood glucose and low or zero blood insulin; a Type 2 diabetic will have high blood glucose and high blood insulin. *Type 2 diabetes, at least in its early stages, can be cured.* Diet changes, a reduction in body fat stores and exercise can control and cure this disorder. Exercise has an "insulin-like" effect on the body, because the demands for glucose as an energy source for the working muscles increase the sensitivity to insulin and facilitate removal of glucose from the blood into the working muscles.

Enlarged fat cells have the opposite effect; they become less sensitive to insulin and don't take up glucose, which is converted to fat and stored. The basic dietary changes involve consuming more complex carbohydrates, reducing sugars and reducing total caloric intake.

You've undoubtedly heard about the "obesity epidemic" going on in our country. Type 2 diabetes is on a parallel rise because of overeating and inactivity. Type 2 diabetes increases the risk of coronary heart disease and of becoming a Type 1 diabetic. Type 1 diabetics have greatly increased risk of kidney failure, blindness and limb amputation.

As the rise in Type 2 diabetes shadows the rise in obesity, the rise in Type 1 diabetes shadows the rise in Type 2 diabetes. This has huge future implications for our healthcare system because of the financial costs of treating those with Type 1 diabetes who have kidney failure and require dialysis treatment or organ transplants.

Remember that Type 1 diabetes is not curable, but it is treatable. A lifestyle with a good diet and exercise and proper medication administration need not lead to negative health consequences. But not doing that will lead to poor health outcomes. The reason a Type 2 diabetic can become a Type 1 diabetic is because the insulin resistance increases with inactivity and body fat accumulation.

Eventually the Beta cells in the pancreas fatigue and start to die off, with an outcome of less insulin production; this is the slide into Type 1 diabetes. It starts with a small insulin injection supplement but eventually no insulin is produced and the individual becomes a Type 1 diabetic. At this stage it's too late to cure.

This particular Type 1 diabetes has nothing to do with a virus or the immune system attacking the Beta cells. For the most part it is a self-indulgent disease due to poor eating habits and inactivity. *This is why it's so important to intervene as early as possible by eating well, maintaining a healthy body weight and engaging in regular exercise.*

PREVENTING OR CONTROLLING DIABETES

Those most likely to develop Type 2 diabetes have a family history of the disease, are overweight, have high triglyceride levels in their blood as well as low levels of HDL cholesterol. Those who have a high level of fat in their belly are also more susceptible.

Most effective in curing Type 2 diabetes are lifestyle changes, including diet and exercise. Strength training also is beneficial to those in the pre-diabetic category as well as those who have it. Strength training increases the volume of muscle while reducing fat. All exercise increases the ability of your body to clear glucose from your blood stream efficiently and decreases insulin resistance.

> Paul, a diabetic, added: "People on Medicare are eligible for free treatment and diabetes education at 'Certified Diabetes Education' centers across the United States. They're usually connected to a hospital. A beginner goes to a series of classes and then is eligible twice a year for free counseling; once a year with a nutritionist and once a year with a diabetes-certified counselor. I've been going for five years and have learned a tremendous amount."

> ### JOE'S BLOOD WORK
>
> For years Joe has used a low dosage, 10 mg, of a statin to control his cholesterol. Then, about two years ago, he found that he was developing Type 2 diabetes and needed to take a medication for that. On the next scheduled tests, the doctor recommended doubling the dosage of the diabetes medication.
>
> A year later the doctor wanted to increase his statin to 40 mg and

again double the dosage of the diabetes medication. The doctor had been urging Joe for some years to start an aggressive exercise program as well as meet with a nutritionist. Joe had not bought into that program but this visit was a wake-up call. They agreed to delay the statin and diabetes medication increases pending the results of his new exercise program.

Joe started riding a recumbent bike at our fitness center three times a week, advancing from twenty to thirty minutes, using the fat-burning program. The next blood work showed a drop in cholesterol but not glucose, the diabetes problem. The discussion with his doctor led to an increased exercise program.

Joe now does seventy minutes on the recumbent bike three times a week, averaging twenty miles per hour. He's dropped ten pounds and two inches around his waist. He consumes more fiber from cereals, vegetables and fruit, plus minimizes his consumption of white potatoes, pasta and red meats. Joe said, "I'm working on The Extended Warranty Program." I think he's planning to be alive and healthy for the long haul.

METABOLIC SYNDROME

Wikipedia defines metabolic syndrome as "a combination of medical disorders that increase the risk of developing cardiovascular disease and diabetes. It affects one in five people, and prevalence increases with age. Some studies estimate the prevalence in the United States to be up to twenty-five percent of the population."

Older people who have large waistlines, high blood pressure and other risk factors also have a higher risk of memory problems. A French study involving over 7,000 participants over the age of sixty-five found that sixteen percent had metabolic syndrome. They were found to be thirteen percent more likely to have problems on a visual memory test.

STROKES

A stroke is a condition in which the blood supply to the brain is interrupted or reduced. This deprives the brain of needed oxygen and blood and brain cells begin to die. A stroke creates an emergency condition that requires immediate medical attention; the sooner the treatment, the better the recovery.

The good news is that the number of deaths from strokes has declined in recent years. Likely reasons are an improvement in monitoring and treating high blood pressure and cholesterol, both big contributors to strokes.

A study of 265 adults, average age of sixty-eight, who had a stroke and were able to walk, found that the top twenty-five percent in terms of exercising regularly were much more likely to suffer a less-severe stroke than those who did little or no exercise prior to their stroke. Physical exercise will also help in recovery from a stroke as well as help to prevent a new one. Talk to your doctor about what exercises you should and shouldn't do.

SURVIVING A STROKE

Another story from Cathy, the director of our SW Florida fitness center: "My mother Emily had a stroke at age eighty . . . she had begun her exercise program at the age of seventy-three at the fitness facility I owned. My dad came and worked out too . . . he was eighty-one.

"Mom worked with one of the personal trainers on staff and my dad did too. I couldn't train either of them because it was hard for them to take direction from me. My dad was wondering when I was going to get a 'real' job.

"The trainer incrementally increased mom's workouts; I think at age seventy-five she could leg press 180 pounds — more than a lot of young desk jocks. She also participated in group exercise classes where she had fun and felt great.

"OK, back to the stroke; because she had been working out and was in good shape at the time of the stroke Emily had complete recovery. Don't get me wrong — she worked hard in both physical and occupational therapy and we hired a personal trainer to come to her home. I constantly challenged her to do more and she would.

"It's all about attitude, persistence — and it goes back to 'the WHY'... When the physical therapist asked what do you want to accomplish, mom said, 'I want to drive again', an aggressive goal. She drives today at age eighty-eight.

"The expectations that you can do more makes most people feel that we haven't given up on them. For my mom's eighty-fifty birthday, my mom, my daughter (who was pregnant with her fourth girl), the other three granddaughters and I did a commercial for Mercy Hospital's Birthing Center . . . four generations. This was an all-day photo shoot in the summer heat and mom said it was the best birthday . . . so much fun. And yes, she stole the show!"

Following are some additional stories of people with other health issues. They're examples of what determined individuals can do.

MARCUS AND HIS KIDNEYS

Marcus, now eighty-eight, is a native of Portland, ME. He's reasonably fit but has never had an active aerobic and strength training program. Recently Marcus was having some balance problems so he went in for a checkup. Blood work determined that he had an elevated kidney function. The doctor, a nephrologist, said that if the numbers went any higher he'd have to go on dialysis.

Marcus started a physical therapy program of strength training and balance exercises to deal with his problems with balance. After two months the results were not only an improvement in his balance but also his kidney function. His doctor was amazed; his GFR, a measure of kidney function, dropped from 4.0 to 2.8.

Marcus has now been asked to participate in a study to determine the effects of a comprehensive fitness program on kidney function. He's motivated to stay around — it's a five-year study.

DEVELOPMENTALLY DISABLED

Ann has a developmentally disabled brother, now fifty-eight. She passed on this story:

"It really came about because I had just read John Ratey's book, *Spark; The Revolutionary New Science of Exercise and the Brain* and thought we ought to present an exercise option to my brother.

"Because of poor balance and coordination, anxiety and overall lack of encouragement, he had never embarked upon any physical activity in his life. Three years ago it was suggested that walking on a treadmill might be a goal he could achieve. Despite doubts all around that he could accomplish this he began walking a few minutes each morning. It's been over three years now and he continues to walk for a half hour, five days a week. When he feels especially anxious he chooses to get back on the treadmill and walk for another session. His sense of accomplishment is such that it's inspired others in his day program to walk on the treadmill as well."

THE FRUSTRATED SWIMMER

Jerry had a stroke in February 2010; this was on top of an existing knee problem, one hip replacement, atrial fibrillation and a shoulder problem that has restricted his ability to swim laps, his favorite exercise. He'd done that for many years.

Despite these problems, Jerry goes to our fitness center five or six days a week. He does strength training exercises using various machines and walks on the treadmill for up to one mile, depending on how his knee is feeling.

Jerry had to be hospitalized twice in the past year for four to five days each time. He learned the reality of how fast muscles will atrophy if they aren't used. He said, "Whether you have limitations or not, develop a program and religiously stick with it. It's amazing how fast you can lose it if you don't use it."

THE BEST MEDICINE

Paul is taking a class at the University of California, Berkeley. The title of the course is "Discovering the Passages of the Third Age" — the period from age fifties to the end. It's being taught by Gail Sheehy, the author of *Passages* and other books.

When he read this chapter he said: "I keep meaning to tell you this. Do you know that laughter is very healthy and may prolong your life?

"In the first Gail Sheehy class she brought in an expert on laughter. This expert also teaches Laughter Yoga. The laughter is more than the laugh one gets from telling jokes; it's the actual act of laughing. The expert showed a video of people awaiting kidney dialysis and doing thirty minutes of laughing before the dialysis. All patients actually had an easier time during the dialysis if they did the laughter before than if they didn't.

"I immediately thought of you and how hard you laugh when I tell you things sometimes. A lot of times I've found myself telling you just to hear you laugh. It's awesome. Keep it up and you may live to seventy-five." (Laughter)

JUDY'S RECOVERY

Two years ago Judy, age sixty-nine, was finding it difficult to breathe properly. She went in for tests and learned that she had what turned out to be a benign tumor in her chest cavity the size of a small melon. The pressure of the tumor was blocking eighty percent of her airway.

This was major surgery requiring a large incision and a long recovery. As soon as she was sufficiently recovered she had two months of daily radiation; it was exhausting. Radiation is cumulative in its debilitation.

Months later Judy was still in pain and had limited use of her right arm. This was disturbing as she's a right-handed artist who lifts reasonably heavy objects; she couldn't do it anymore. Her doctor confirmed that lifting anything bigger than a teacup was likely to be a continuing problem so he prescribed physical therapy.

After only three weeks of physical therapy the muscles on her right side began to function again. The physical therapist said, "You're getting your muscle memory back." Also, she experienced a ninety percent reduction in pain, a huge difference for her.

This was Judy's awakening. She acquired a treadmill for aerobics and weights for strength training. She's now working out regularly in her home and plans to continue the physical therapy for several more months. Of course, she's also back to her work as an artist.

OVERCOMING ADVERSITY

There's a clear pattern you can see in the stories in this chapter — Cathy recovering from her accident, Bob avoiding braces and canes, Stu arresting his Parkinson's, yours truly overcoming the pain of a herniated disc without surgery.

Each individual had their mind overcome their body — they took action that overcame their physical problems. Some had done little or no organized exercise before but that didn't stop them from getting out of their comfort zone and taking charge of their body. They exhibited the motivation and discipline needed to change their life.

If they can do it, you can, too.

LET'S REVIEW

- Health problems can be overcome. The stories in this chapter are living proof of that.

- If you have any of the health issues discussed, be sure to solicit the advice of your doctor prior to undertaking a serious exercise program.

- If you don't have any of the problems discussed in this chapter, an excellent way to maintain that is to implement a program of regular exercise and healthy eating.

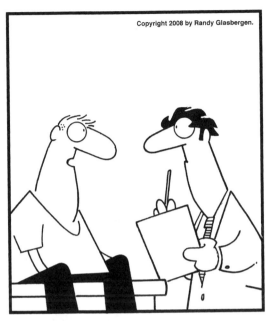

Copyright 2008 by Randy Glasbergen.

"If I'm digging my grave with a fork and spoon, wouldn't that burn a lot of calories?"

CHAPTER TEN — HEALTHY EATING

"Those who think they have no time for healthy eating will sooner or later have to find time for illness." — Edward Stanley, 1826–1893

HERE'S WHAT'S COMING

- Cholesterol and lipoproteins — what do you need to know?
- Fats — what should you avoid and why?
- Why is writing down what you eat — at least for awhile — valuable?
- What does fiber intake have to do with longevity?
- Water, salt and potassium — how much do you need?
- Sugar — why should you watch how much you eat?
- Whole grains — how much is enough?
- Servings — all servings are not created equal. How do you measure a serving?

WHAT'S THE MESSAGE?

Syms, a clothing store chain, is famous for their slogan, "An Educated Consumer Is Our Best Customer." The goal in this chapter is to help you become an Educated Consumer.

More knowledge about food will enable you to make better choices about what you do and don't eat. There's action that you can take — like writing down what you eat and learning how many calories and how much of carbohydrates, protein and fat are in your normal diet. The goal is for more information to lead to better decisions.

FOUR BOWLING BALLS

A man's bowling ball weighs sixteen pounds. Four equals sixty-four pounds. Joe lost weight the equivalent of four and a half bowling balls in fifteen months.

Joe, seventy-four, has worked at the beach club of our SW Florida community since 2001. Back then he weighed 279 pounds; he's five feet four inches tall. His weight per inch of height was off the charts.

In February 2004, as a result of making some eating changes, he was down to 239 pounds. This is what he weighed in January 2009, when he decided enough was enough; time to get serious. As Joe said, "You gotta make up your mind to do it; nobody can do it for you. We all know what to do; it's just deciding to do it."

So what did he do? He kicked junk out of the house. If there was a half-gallon of ice cream in the freezer, he'd eat it — in one sitting. He'd do the same with a dozen chocolate chip cookies. Joe decided that if he couldn't see it, he wouldn't eat it. The rule today is — no junk in the house, plus Joe chooses to not eat white bread, white potatoes and processed foods.

Joe has lots of color in his diet from vegetables and fruit. Joe also eats a lot of fish, chicken and pork. He'll have red meat maybe once a month. *Joe didn't go on a diet, he made a lifestyle change.* Diets are temporary, life changes can be permanent. His wife saw what happened to Joe and signed up for the program. She's lost forty-five pounds, with no pressure from Joe. She made up her mind also.

Today Joe weighs 169 pounds and is mighty proud of it, as he should be. He does some walking and now we'll try to get him doing some regular fitness exercises. He's on a roll, so why not?

Joe's had sleep apnea for fifteen years and has been sleeping with an oxygen mask. Recently he was having more than his usual trouble sleeping and learned that, as a result of his weight loss, he needed fifty percent less oxygen. Getting too much oxygen was keeping him awake.

It's likely that Joe's increased both the length of his life and the quality of life he'll enjoy for years to come.

MIKE'S YO-YO

I met Mike on a ride with our local bike club in Bucks County, PA. He's fifty-one years old, five feet nine inches tall. In December 2002, he weighed in at 224 pounds. He'd spent more than a dozen years on yo-yo diets; he'd lose it and put it right back on.

He joined Weight Watchers and started exercising by running forty-five minutes five days a week. In a few months he developed a problem with his feet and found running painful. A friend suggested cycling which he initially rejected; he said, "Cycling's for wimps." But, he dusted off his bike and started cycling on a path nearby plus continued running, albeit painfully.

Within six months of Weight Watchers, running and cycling, Mike had dropped fifty pounds. He lost an additional ten the next year and has maintained that weight ever since. He began to cycle more. He bought a good bike and rode his first century — a hundred-mile ride — in 2004.

Six years ago he learned about our local bike club, started riding with a group and found it very motivational. He started tracking his mileage; from January 2006 to the end of 2009, he rode 33,700 miles, an average of over 8,400 miles per year. Understand he's fifty-one, works full-time and it's cold in Bucks County in the winter. He says there are two conditions in which he doesn't ride outdoors in the winter — snow and ice. Temperature is not an issue as he and some friends ride in ten-degree weather.

Mike eats healthy food but occasionally rewards himself with some chocolate chip cookies and his favorite ice cream. He drinks lots of water and says he hasn't had a soda for seven years. He knows that as long as he exercises as he does now he will keep the weight off. As he said, "The sport of cycling has changed my life."

Mike's a life member of Weight Watchers and weighs in once a month. He's made the lifestyle changes that will keep him healthy.

Let's talk about some information that's helpful for you to know about yourself as well as what you choose to eat and drink. This is information about your blood content — cholesterol and lipoproteins — the different types of fat and what's a good mix of carbohydrates, protein and fat in your diet.

CHOLESTEROL AND LIPOPROTEINS

Cholesterol is not all bad — it's a necessary part of our body chemistry. We get it from two sources; our body produces it in our liver, which accounts for about seventy-five percent of what we have, and the other twenty-five percent comes from what we eat. It's only found in the animal foods we consume.

All cholesterol is combined with proteins and phosphate to make lipoproteins. Lipoproteins are the carriers for fat and cholesterol in our bloodstream. Since blood is a water-based medium, it's necessary to have a substance that can transport fat and cholesterol (which has solubility characteristics similar to fat) in the bloodstream. There are four types of lipoproteins:

Chylomicrons — These transport dietary cholesterol to the liver for processing and are the dominant type of lipoprotein following a fatty meal.

VLDL (Very Low Density Lipoprotein) — After the fat has been removed by the liver, this is the remnant of the chylomicron.

LDL (Low-Density Lipoprotein) — This is formed in the liver and is the primary carrier of cholesterol to the cells of the body. It's the primary source of buildup of fatty deposits and cholesterol in the arteries, especially the coronary arteries. This is the BAD cholesterol and the more that's in your blood, the greater your chance of coronary heart disease.

HDL (High-Density Lipoprotein) — This is the GOOD cholesterol. It carries cholesterol from parts of the body to the liver, where it's removed from the body. HDL helps the body get rid of cholesterol, thereby reducing the buildup in arteries. The higher one's HDL, the better.

Triglycerides — Another form of fat in our body is a triglyceride. It consists of three fatty acid molecules attached to a sugar alcohol called glycerol. Well over ninety percent of the fat in our body is in the form of triglycerides, including all that's stored in our fat cells. Lipoproteins transport most fat in the form of triglycerides. A high triglyceride number is linked to coronary artery disease in some people.

THE NUMBERS

Cholesterol is measured in milligrams (mg) per deciliter (dl) of blood. A total cholesterol reading of 200 mg/dl or less is ideal.

LDL — Seventy mg/dl measurement or less is good for individuals with a high risk of heart disease based on family history, weight, etc. While 100 to 130 is OK for everyone else, we'd all like to be below 100. The recommendation for anyone who has coronary artery disease (CAD) is a reading below seventy.

HDL — Sixty mg/dl or more is terrific. A reading below forty for men and fifty for men is not good. If you're in this range, talk to your doctor.

Triglycerides — Normal is an mg/dl less than 150; high is 200 to 499 and very high is over 500.

TRIGLYCERIDES AND STROKES

I was listening to NPR recently and heard a discussion of the role of triglycerides in strokes. They reported on a twenty-year study in Denmark of 16,000 individuals. The study was designed to determine the role of cholesterol and triglycerides in strokes. During that period 1,600 of those in the study died of strokes.

The results showed that high triglycerides were a major factor in strokes. In fact, for women high cholesterol was not a significant factor but high triglycerides were. The study was published in the *Annals of Internal Medicine*.

FAT: THE GOOD, THE BAD, THE UGLY

There's fat and there's fat; we need some of it in our diet, just not too much and especially not too much of the wrong kind. The issues are both quantity and quality. Fat has nine calories per gram versus four for protein and carbohydrates, so it's a concentrated source of energy. Fat helps the absorption of the fat soluble vitamins A, D, E and K. Fat is a carrier of flavor in food; food wouldn't taste very good without it.

GOOD FATS

Monounsaturated Fats — Think nuts: peanuts, cashews, almonds and pistachios, for example. Olive oil and canola oil are also good sources, as are avocados. The good news is that these guys can actually lower LDL as well as increase HDL in our blood. HDL is what we want more of in our blood.

Polyunsaturated Fats — Seafood like salmon and fish oil have this, also corn, soy, safflower and sunflower oils. They can lower LDL, a good thing, but too much can also lower HDL, not a good thing.

Omega-3 Fatty Acids — These are a "must-have," as our body doesn't produce them. Good sources are cold-water fish, such as salmon, halibut and tuna, plus some nuts, like walnuts. They play a big role in brain function as well as normal growth and development. Many of us take a fish oil tablet twice a day to ensure a good supply.

In the 1970s researchers studied the Greenland Inuit tribe. They eat lots of fat via seafood but have virtually no cardiovascular disease. The high level of Omega-3 fatty acids they consume was the reason.

BAD FATS

Saturated fats — Think animals; meat and dairy products are easy to remember. Beef, cheese and eggs are good examples. Some plants are sources also, like palm oil and palm kernel oil; these are often found in baked goods and chips.

What's wrong with saturated fats? Simple; they're the culprits that contribute to the clogging of our arteries and raise our LDL level. It's important to minimize the consumption of saturated fats.

UGLY FATS

Trans Fats or Hydrogenated Fats — Hydrogenation is the process of treating unsaturated fats with hydrogen to make them saturated. They then take on the characteristics of saturated fat, including increased stability. The result is the formation of trans fats. Why do this? Because products treated with hydrogenated fats have a longer shelf life. Good examples are cookies, cakes, French fries and donuts.

If the label of a product says it contains hydrogenated oil or partially hydrogenated oil, it contains trans fats. Manufacturers are now required to list trans fat content on food labels. The same problem exists with trans fats as with saturated fats — they're artery cloggers.

You need to check the labels carefully for these. The requirement to list trans fats is in force if it has over .5 grams of trans fats. Some have circumvented this issue by simply lowering the serving size so that a serving falls below this number.

DOM'S DIET

A few months ago Dom and I had lunch. He said, "I eat red meat nearly every day, but I don't eat much with lots of marbled fat. Is anything wrong with that?" Dom is in his early forties.

Let's compare a few dinner entrees that Dom might choose from. All of the numbers shown are in grams. Fat has nine calories per gram while protein and carbohydrates have four.

Dinners		Calories	Carbs	Protein	Fat	Sat Fat	Fiber	Sugar
Filet Mignon	6 oz	370	0	46	18	8	0	0
Big Mac w/Cheese	7 oz	540	47	25	30	10	3	8
Halibut	6 oz	223	0	42	5	1	0	0
Chicken Breast	6 oz	248	0	47	6	1	0	0

Every night that Dom eats filet mignon he digests 160 calories of fat, of which fifty are saturated fat. Halibut, by comparison, contains about thirty calories of fat with almost no saturated fat. A chicken dinner is very similar. Four nights a week of chicken or fish versus filet mignon would reduce his fat intake by over 500 calories, of which 180 would be saturated fat. The Big Mac with Cheese? We won't even go there.

> Dom, I think you'd best develop a liking for more fish and chicken.
> Your health would definitely benefit from eating less saturated fat.

WRITE IT DOWN

I remember talking to a friend after he'd made a hole-in-one playing golf. He said, "It's not that hard." What's not that hard, you ask? The act of writing down what you eat so that you know how much you're eating in total calories, carbohydrates, protein, fat, etc. Writing it down sounds much harder than it is.

I recently signed up for a pilot program at our Florida fitness center during which a dozen of us will keep detailed records of our eating and exercise habits. While I keep records of exercise, I haven't kept similar records of my food and drink. It's been a very enlightening experience.

Following is a chart that summarizes some items for breakfast, lunch and dinner. You can obtain data from various books as well as the USDA Food and Nutrition Center. The easy way to access this site is to Google "USDA Food Database." While the USDA site is very complete, it's also a bit complex to use.

Another site that's easy to use is "nutritiondata.self.com." You enter the food item and it generates a food label with the information. They state on their site that the data is taken from the USDA database.

Food labels on items you buy packaged are an easy source. An inexpensive, very complete paperback book is *The Complete Book of Food Counts* by Corinne T. Netzer. A very thorough book is *Bowe's and Church's Food Values of Portions Commonly Used* by Pennington and Spungen. The 2011 edition is expensive but used copies of the previous edition are available at a low price.

The big awakening for me was the cocktail hour. If I drink two five-ounce glasses of wine plus eat a fair amount of cashews or walnuts (translation: three to four ounces), I can easily consume 800 calories. About a third of those are "empty calories" in the form of alcohol, which have no redeeming value. Also, drinking more tends to lead to our "dropping our guard" and eating more, a double whammy.

> Roger added: "Some would question this: alcohol elevates HDL, reduces the stress response and facilitates social interaction. Moderation is the key." Good points, Roger; I personally don't plan to eliminate all alcohol, just to exercise more moderation.

If I limit my consumption of empty calories to one five-ounce glass versus two and have just one ounce of nuts, I cut the total by at least fifty percent. Those 400 hundred calories total 2,800 for a week, 145,000 per year; that's over forty pounds of potential fat.

Breakfast	Quantity	Calories	Carbs	Protein	Fat	Sat Fat	Fiber	Sugar
Cantaloupe	¼	70	16	2	0	0	2	16
Blueberries	½ cup	57	15	1	0	0	2	10
Strawberries	½ cup	32	8	1	1	0	2	5
Banana	1	105	27	1	0	0	3	14
Oatmeal	½ cup	150	27	5	3	0	4	1
Apple (In Sauce)	½ cup	56	15	0	0	0	3	12
Raisins	1.5 oz	129	25	1	0	0	2	25
Milk – Skim	1 cup	100	19	13	0	0	0	19
Apple Juice	½ cup	46	11	0	0	0	0	10
Total		745	163	24	4	0	18	112

Lunch	Quantity	Calories	Carbs	Protein	Fat	Sat Fat	Fiber	Sugar
Turkey Breast	6 oz	200	0	40	1	0	0	0
Swiss Cheese	1 slc	40	1	3	1	1	0	0
Honey Mustard	2 tsp	20	4	0	0	0	0	2
Health Nut Bread	2	240	42	10	4	0	4	6
Sweet Gherkins Pickles	4	70	16	0	0	0	0	14
Potato Chips – Baked	1 oz	110	23	2	2	0	2	2
Total		680	86	55	8	1	6	24

Cocktails – Options	Quantity	Calories	Carbs	Protein	Fat	Sat Fat	Fiber	Sugar
Wine	10 oz	250	11	0	0	0	0	0
Gin and Tonic – 2 oz gin	1	150	12	0	0	0	0	12
Cashews	1 oz	160	0	5	12	4	1	2
Walnuts	1 oz	180	4	4	18	2	2	1
Snacks	1 cup	240	0	4	8	2	2	4
Total		980	27	13	38	8	5	19

Dinners	Quantity	Calories	Carbs	Protein	Fat	Sat Fat	Fiber	Sugar
Filet Mignon	6 oz	360	0	48	18	6	0	0
Baked Potato	1	145	34	3	0	0	2	3
Green Beans	1 cup	44	10	2	1	0	4	2
Ice Cream Sandwich – Low-Fat	1	140	30	4	2	1	3	15
Total		**689**	**74**	**57**	**21**	**7**	**9**	**20**
Chicken Breast	6 oz	248	0	47	6	1	0	0
Sweet Potato	1 large	162	37	4	1	0	6	15
Mixed Vegetables	1 cup	50	11	2	0	0	2	3
Ice Cream Sandwich – Low-Fat	1	140	30	4	2	1	3	15
Total		**600**	**78**	**57**	**9**	**2**	**11**	**33**
Halibut	6 oz	189	0	38	3	1	0	0
Brown Rice	1 cup	216	45	5	2	1	4	1
Broccoli	2 spears	26	5	2	0	0	2	1
Ice Cream Sandwich – Low-Fat	1	140	30	4	2	1	3	15
Total		**571**	**80**	**49**	**7**	**3**	**9**	**17**

PERSISTENCE PAYS

Neale, a reviewer from the beginning, read a number of chapters multiple times. His story:

"Your book has had a profound effect on my wellness, far beyond what I imagined when I first began to read it as you were cranking out the drafts.

"I've always enjoyed exercise in various forms, from hiking to cross-country and alpine skiing to occasional weight lifting. Being moderately active, I never thought I had a weight problem. When I first began to read your book last fall, I was somewhat surprised to discover that my 195 pounds placed me over the edge of the limit of the "acceptable range" of 185 pounds for my 6'1" height. That got my attention.

"Then I read the chapter on aerobics. The section on interval training brought back memories of training sessions for track (half-mile and one-mile runs) in high school, and I decided to put some intervals into my workout routine. Very quickly my level of fitness improved. This improvement spurred me on to increase the number of workouts I did per week from three to four to four to five. Then I stepped up the intensity a few notches.

"After I read the chapter on nutrition I began to pay more attention to what I was eating. I made a few small changes in my diet: cut breakfast English muffins from two to one and substituted a spoonful of yogurt for a pat or two of butter on the muffin. My weight stayed the same. Then I cut afternoon cocktail-hour glasses of wine from two to one and occasionally none. Still nothing happened . . . for awhile.

"Suddenly, one day my weight dropped from 195 down to 192. I stepped up the workouts a notch. A couple of weeks later the scales tipped at 186. I started eating slightly smaller portions, especially at dinner, and a few weeks after that the scale hit 180. Occasionally I have a dip below 180 or rise to 185, but generally I can stay in the 180–185 range without difficulty. This is a very happy outcome for me.

"Note that these changes didn't occur in a smooth, linear fashion — the pattern was choppy. No change for long periods, punctuated by periods of rapid but irregular change. The only thing that stayed relatively consistent was my pattern of exercise and then, later, the closer 'management' of my diet. The pattern of my exercise did change gradually from a moderate level in the beginning to a more frequent and more intense level now.

"The key words are 'gradual' and 'consistent.' Perhaps a better word would be 'persistent.' I didn't give up. I kept going, even when nothing seemed to be happening. But, as you point out in the book, in terms of my physiology things were definitely happening. Because of the contextual understanding provided by your book I was able to 'keep the faith,' and stick to the program. As a result, very positive changes have occurred. I remain forever grateful that your book has provided the stimulation and inspiration to help me make positive changes in my lifestyle."

HOW MUCH OF EACH?

What's a good mix? The USDA recommends forty-five percent to sixty-five percent of daily calories be from carbohydrates, twenty-five percent to thirty-five percent from protein and twenty percent to thirty-five percent from fats. If you're more active — doing serious strength training, for example — various sources recommend a mix of fifty percent carbohydrates, thirty percent proteins and twenty percent fat. If you're somewhere in that range and enjoying an active life via exercise, you'll be fine.

JUST DON'T BUY IT

What's the easy way to be sure you don't eat something? You know the answer — don't allow it in the house. My wife Deb and I have cut out a number of items using this simple solution.

I love frozen yogurt in a waffle cone after dinner. If it's in the house, I'll eat it and never give it a thought; Deb will, too. She was counting up her calories and asked me not to buy the yogurt or cones anymore. I reluctantly agreed but, within a week, I was out of the habit. Instead, I buy a low-fat ice cream sandwich that's 100 calories versus about 500 for the yogurt and cone.

FIBER AND LONGEVITY

On February 14, 2011, researchers from the U.S. National Cancer Institute reported that eating a diet rich in fiber may reduce your risk of dying from heart disease, respiratory disease or any other cause by twenty-two percent.

This study involved over 388,000 men and women — 219,000 men and 169,000 women — who, in 1995 and 1996, filled out a detailed questionnaire asking about their diet. The amount of fiber eaten by those in the study ranged from thirteen to twenty-nine grams per day for men and from eleven to twenty-six grams per day for women.

Over the nine years of follow-up, 20,126 men and 11,330 women died. The researchers found that the men and women who ate the most fiber were twenty-two percent less likely to die over the nine-year period than those who ate the least amount of fiber.

Also, the risk of cardiovascular and respiratory disease was cut by twenty-four percent to fifty-six percent among the men who ate the most fiber and reduced by thirty-four percent to fifty-nine percent among the women who ate the most fiber. Fiber from grains, but not from fruits, was the most beneficial in reducing the risk of premature death.

Lead researcher Yikung Park said, "Prior studies have focused on the relationship between fiber intake and cardiovascular disease, but few have examined the link between dietary fiber and risk of death from any cause. Our analysis adds to the literature and suggests dietary fiber intake is associated with decreased likelihood of death."

Samantha Heller at the Center for Cancer Care at Griffin Hospital in Derby, CT, said, "Wouldn't it be great if people took the simple step of adding healthy, high-fiber foods to their diets and dodged very scary and serious diseases such as cardiovascular disease, cancer and diabetes?"

The recommended daily fiber intake for those over fifty was thirty grams for men and twenty-one grams for women. For perspective, a half-cup of All-Bran is equal to ten grams of fiber.

GOOD FIBER SOURCES

Eating an adequate amount of fiber is relatively easy; it just takes a bit of knowledge and some changes in eating habits. Let's review some good sources.

Fruits — Review the summary of breakfast fruits on page 223. You can easily consume seven to ten grams of fiber at breakfast.

Breads — There are seven grams of fiber in a whole wheat bagel and four grams in two slices of Health Nut Bread. The whole wheat bagel has a total of forty-nine grams of carbohydrates and seven grams of sugar, so factor those in also. The two slices of Health Nut Bread have twenty-one grams of carbohydrates, less than half of the bagel, plus only three grams of sugar. Choose breads that say "whole wheat" or "whole grains."

Cereals — Many breakfast cereals are high in fiber, but be sure to check the sugar and sodium content. Try other whole grains like buckwheat groats, quinoa, barley and farro. You can look them up online. Oatmeal has four grams in a one-half cup.

Vegetables — They're loaded with fiber. Green beans have four grams of fiber in a one-cup serving, for example, as does broccoli. A cup of carrots has almost seven grams. One cup of whole wheat pasta also has four grams. Brown rice has over five grams of fiber in a one-half cup.

Frequently, when foods are processed, the fiber is removed. Avoid foods made from white flour such as white bread, pizza and regular pasta. If you're uncertain as to whether you're getting enough fiber consider taking a dietary supplement such as Citrucel or Metamucil, which provide four to six grams of fiber mixed in an eight-ounce glass of water.

YOUR BRAIN ON FOOD

What and how much you eat have a significant impact on the health of your brain as well as the rest of your body. A long-term study of 1,500 adults found those who were obese were twice as likely to develop dementia in later life. A high intake of saturated fat and cholesterol clogs the arteries and is associated with a higher risk of Alzheimer's.

Dark-skinned fruits and vegetables have the highest concentration of antioxidants, which are good for you. Examples are eggplant, spinach, red bell peppers, apples, blueberries, raisins, plums, cranberries and cherries. Eat them with the skin for maximum benefit.

Cold-water fish have more omega-3 fatty acids, and are also good for you — halibut, mackerel, salmon, trout and tuna. Nuts such as almonds, pecans and walnuts provide vitamin E, an antioxidant.

WATER, SALT AND POTASSIUM

Water — Most of us drink plenty of water by simply drinking when we're thirsty. The old recommendation that we consume eight glasses per day has been proven to be false. We obtain water from a variety of sources in addition to what we drink directly: coffee, tea, fruits, vegetables and soft drinks, for example. We may not need eight glasses per day, but keeping well hydrated is important for your body.

Salt is a necessary ingredient in our life — the problem is the quantity. Most of us consume much more salt than our bodies need. A normal level of daily salt intake is 1,100 to 3,300 mg, but many of us have much more than that. The problem with higher levels is that excess salt causes your body to retain more water to dilute the salt.

Excess salt increases the fluid around your cells and in your blood vessels. This leads to increased pressure on all your arteries, capillaries and veins, and consequent blood pressure and puts more demands on your heart. As a result, your heart has to work harder to pump the blood in the blood vessels, which are compressed by the water retention.

Some South American Indians used to get along just fine with 200 mg per day. Keep in mind that your body will adapt, as best it can, to greater or lesser quantities of dietary salt. When salt intake is reduced the kidneys will conserve salt and reduce elimination. When salt is high in the diet, the kidneys will do the opposite. But chronic high salt intake will exceed the capacity of the kidneys to eliminate the salt and the extra salt will be retained, leading to greater water retention and the potential for hypertension.

A Harvard Medical School Special Health Report, "Hypertension — Controlling the 'Silent Killer'" provides an excellent list of twenty strategies for reducing salt input. It's difficult to determine how much salt you are ingesting at any given time. The best way to exercise some degree of control is to limit consumption of processed foods, not use salt at the table and reduce the amount of salt in meals while preparing them. Look at the sodium content of products you eat regularly; it's shown on the nutrition facts label.

Potassium is a mineral that plays a big role in the function of cells, tissues and organs in the body. It's very important in the function of our heart and in muscular contraction. If you eat a diet with lots of whole grains, fruits and vegetables you're likely to have a higher level of potassium in your system. Bananas and potatoes have lots of potassium; dairy and meat products also are a good source.

There have been some links of low potassium with high blood pressure and a higher risk of stroke. Note that potassium supplements don't seem to have the same benefits as potassium in food.

WHAT ABOUT SUGAR?

First of all, sugar is sugar; it doesn't matter whether it's the white out of the five-pound bag, honey or maple syrup. They're all simple sugars. Over the last twenty years we've increased the average sugar consumption by twenty-six pounds to 135 pounds per year — that's about two and a half pounds per week. This compares to five pounds per year per person in the late nineteenth century.

The big issue is not the teaspoon in your morning coffee — fifteen calories — it's the sugar we don't see in donuts, processed foods and soft drinks. The typical adult consumes about 350 calories of sugar a day — approximately 10,000 calories per month, or almost three pounds. That translates into thirty-six pounds of fat per year.

The *Journal of the American Medical Association* reported that those who consume the largest amount of sugar have higher triglycerides and lower HDL — the good cholesterol. Both contribute to a higher risk of heart disease. Those who ate the least had the lowest triglycerides and highest HDL.

While sugar doesn't cause type 2 diabetes directly, those who consume lots of sugar tend to be overweight or obese. They are much stronger candidates to get type 2 diabetes. Sugar also raises insulin levels, which depresses the immune system. We like to keep our immune system active in order to avoid health problems.

What's a person to do? Limit consumption of foods and drinks that are obviously high in sugar content. If you're unsure, look at the label. A product with fifty grams of sugar has 200 empty calories.

THE GOOD AND BAD OF PROCESSED FOODS

Processed foods are simply foods that have been modified from their natural state. Examples are foods processed by freezing, canning, refrigeration, dehydration and with substances added like chemicals, preservatives, vitamins, salts, etc.

Many foods that have been processed are good for us. Milk that we buy in a store, for example, has been pasteurized and homogenized. We benefit from frozen vegetables as the nutrients are retained and we can eat them year-round. Fruit juices are another healthy example.

The problem is with the ingestion of processed foods that contain lots of sodium, trans fats, saturated fats and sugar. How do you know the difference? Read the labels. Examples of processed food to limit or avoid are potato chips and other snacks, breads and pastas made with refined white flour versus whole grains, canned foods loaded with sodium and/or fat and breakfast cereals with lots of sugar.

You may say, "Harry, that's all fine and good, but I'm a busy man or woman. I don't have time to read every label of every item when I go shopping." Fair enough;

but what about reading a few each time? Begin with some that are likely suspects like snacks. Find out what's in them in terms of fats, sodium and sugar. Do the same with any breakfast cereal.

It doesn't take much thought to know which foods are high in sugar and salt. Are they sweet? Are they salty? Once you pay attention to those foods, start to read the labels of other foods. A few minutes of diligence is likely to lead to you becoming a more educated consumer.

WHAT ABOUT WHOLE GRAINS?

The new *Dietary Guidelines for Americans 2010* published by the U.S. Agriculture and Health and Human Services Departments are that we should consume at least half of the recommended six servings of grains daily as whole grains versus refined grains. Whole grains include barley, corn, including whole corn meal and popcorn, oats, brown or colored rice, rye, wheat and wild rice. If you have a snack of popcorn without butter, that's a whole grain.

One of the best ways to be sure you eat whole grains is with breakfast cereal, but read the labels carefully. Some have a lot more of whole grains than others, plus some are loaded with sugar. If you consume about 2,000 calories per day you should eat about fifty grams or 200 calories each of whole grains and refined grains. To put that in perspective, you can get about sixteen grams from a slice of bread or a cup of cereal. Whole wheat pasta and brown rice are other good sources.

WHAT ABOUT SNACKS?

For years I've heard that eating lots of small meals — snacking between the normal breakfast, lunch and dinner — is a good idea, but I never understood why. It turns out that there are two good reasons:

1. Maintain energy. Ever have that feeling of running out of gas in the middle of the morning or afternoon? We all have. We had a meal a few hours ago, have digested it, used up much of the energy provided and now have a gas tank approaching empty. We need some fuel.

2. Avoid gorging at the next meal. If we resist the urge to have something to provide energy we'll be famished at the next meal and run the risk of overeating.

There are snacks and there are snacks, and they aren't created equally. Some good choices are fresh fruit, like an apple or banana, air-popped popcorn, which is very filling, cashews, walnuts or peanuts, in a small quantity, or vegetables like carrots or steamed broccoli. The nuts have fat but it's monounsaturated, the best kind. Just don't eat too many of them as they're high in calories.

EAT LIKE A GREEK

We've known for years that the Mediterranean diet reduces mortality from cardiovascular disease and cancer. A recent analysis of data from fifty different studies and over 500,000 participants found an over thirty percent reduction in metabolic syndrome for those who live the Mediterranean lifestyle.

Metabolic syndrome is a confluence of a number of health problems — a waist of over forty inches for men and thirty-five inches for women, high blood pressure and blood sugar, low levels of HDL cholesterol and high levels of triglycerides.

The Mediterranean diet — actually a lifestyle, not a diet — has lots of olive oil, whole-grain cereals, fruits and vegetables and fish. There's very little consumption of animal fat.

Dr. Elizabeth Jackson, a cardiologist at the University of Michigan, said, "When people are able to make improvements through diet, they are preventing the need in the future to go on medication."

Sue D read this chapter and said: "Thank you for sending the draft of your latest chapter and please forgive me for not responding sooner. My Dad, age eighty-nine, fell in his condo last week and hit his head. Fortunately, the EMTs took him to the emergency room where they did a CAT scan of the head, stitched him up and released him.

"I attribute no broken bones or further injury to the wonderful shape my father keeps himself in. He walks about a mile every day and eats fruits, vegetables and all the things in your chapter every day."

WHAT'S A SERVING?

All servings aren't created equal. A serving of broccoli, for example, looks nothing like a serving of meat or fish. So how do we know whether we have one serving or maybe much more?

One of the better websites for useful information is WebMD. They provide pictures of the portion size for various foods. Some examples of a serving of various foods:

- One small baked potato = one computer mouse
- One and a half ounces of cheese = three dice
- One cup of apple = one baseball
- One-fourth cup of almonds = one golf ball
- Three ounces of cooked fish = a checkbook
- Two and a half ounces of meat = two-thirds of a deck of cards

Check their website for more information. While I rarely read a book with the word "diet" in the title, I made an exception with *The Mayo Clinic Diet: Eat Well, Enjoy Life, Lose Weight* by a team at the Mayo Clinic. I find it to be a very useful book for practical ideas about healthy eating, including a chart of serving sizes on page seventy-three.

Knowing serving sizes is an important step in healthy eating. Knowing that a tablespoon of cashews — about six nuts — contains almost fifty calories may motivate you to think about just how many cashews you should eat at one sitting.

WHAT'S A SERVING SIZE?

Ever look at a label and think "This is OK, it's only one hundred calories, thirty of which are fat." Later you notice that the calorie count is for about one-third of what you normally consume of that item at one sitting. You neglected to look at the section "Amount per serving."

My wife Deb and I craved some ice cream recently, an item we don't keep in our home. I bought a half gallon of "Edy's Slow Churn Rich and Creamy" which had on the label – "one-third less calories, one-half less fat." There are 130 calories per serving, of which fifty are from fat. When I got home I noticed that a serving is one-quarter of a cup. I ate more than that when I was six years old.

Another good example is peanut butter, which is healthy for a snack or sandwich. The total calories per serving are 190, of which 130 are fat. The serving size is two tablespoons. Most of us likely use four or five tablespoons in a sandwich; that's 800 to 1,000 calories, of which 500 to 800 are fat. Take the time to read the label and understand what you're consuming.

KNOWLEDGE IS POWER

Many of us are creatures of habit. Much of the food we eat on a regular basis falls into a narrow range. It's relatively easy to calculate how many calories we're consuming from our normal breakfasts and lunches. This becomes a one-time activity. You can summarize, as I did earlier in this chapter, your consumption in calories, carbohydrates, fat, etc. You can then do some examples of various dinners eaten at home or in a restaurant.

This activity creates what I call "The Power of Awareness." If you know that those chocolate chip cookies have 300 calories per cookie, mostly fat, and you know that based on what you've eaten that day and the exercise you've done (or haven't done) that they'll put you in the position of adding stored fat, you're less likely to eat them.

I mentioned that a dozen of us are in a program at our fitness center where we are recording eating and exercise information. We're using a device called an "Exerspy" that tracks the number of calories we burn daily, including during sleep hours. We've reached a very high level of awareness as a result of having this information.

Recently four of us were having lunch after golf; three are in this program. All three of us had a bowl of soup plus crackers or a whole-wheat roll. In prior weeks someone would bring over a plate of cookies and we'd all have one or even two. None of us have had a cookie since we started the program. The fourth player has followed the lead of the pack; no cookies for him either.

THE DEVIL'S IN THE DETAILS

Jane Brody wrote an article for *The New York Times* entitled "Still Counting Calories? Your Weight-Loss Plan May Be Outdated." She summarizes data from research by five nutrition and public health experts at Harvard.

What makes this research so meaningful is that it's based on data from over 120,000 well-educated men and women over a period of twelve to twenty years. The participants, all healthcare professionals, were healthy and not obese at the beginning.

Some of the results:

• The average participant gained almost a pound per year for an average total gain of twenty pounds in twenty years. People don't become overweight overnight; it's done slowly, like Chinese torture.

- While physical activity helped, those who were active but ignored what they ate gained weight. As one of the doctors said, "Physical activity in the United States is poor, but diet is even worse."

- What we eat matters. Another doctor said, "There are good foods and bad foods, and the advice should be to eat the good foods more and the bad foods less."

- What foods led to the most gain? French fries were at the top, followed by potato chips, sugar-sweetened drinks, red meats and processed meats, other forms of potatoes and fried foods, butter, fruit juice and desserts. No big surprises here.

- How about the "good guys"? That would be fruits, vegetables and whole grains. Participants who ate more yogurt lost almost a pound every four years. Nuts, including peanut butter, were a positive contributor to weight loss also.

- Dairy products, whether low-fat milk or full-fat milk and cheese, had a neutral effect on weight.

- Those who watched more television gained more weight, likely due to the food ads and snacking while watching. Those who drank one glass of wine per day were fine, but larger amounts and other forms of alcohol led to weight gain.

- An interesting fact: we've talked about resting metabolic rate (RMR), the number of calories burned at rest. RMR decreased after consumption of refined grains but stayed constant after eating whole grains.

A CLASSIC CASE

A friend recently sent me an email she'd received from the restaurant chain, Chick-fil-it. It describes their new offering, a hand-spun banana milkshake. The ad says, "For a limited time, enjoy fresh bananas, vanilla wafers and a splash of vanilla in a delicious, sippable dessert."

Here are the numbers:

	<u>Small</u>	<u>Large</u>
Calories	780	1,010
Fat	24g (216 Calories)	31g (279 Calories)
Saturated Fat	12g (108 Calories)	15g (135 Calories)
Sugars	104g	135g
Sodium	440mg	580mg
Carbohydrates	131g	173g
Protein	22g	30g
Fiber	1g	1g
Cholesterol	65mg	85mg

The total calories in the large milkshake represent about fifty percent of what many individuals should consume — all day. The small is about forty percent. Almost thirty percent of those calories are fat and half of those are saturated fat.

Like I said — knowledge is power.

AN ACTION PLAN

Maureen, in her fifties, read this chapter and said: "Most people know about nutrition, especially if they are reading a fitness/lifestyle book. Counting and listing calories was an eye-opener. I'm sure if we listed everything we put in our mouths we would eat less. Portion control and eating slowly is huge. Conscious eating — not while doing something else or even thinking about something else — is important.

"I went to the gynecologist last week. I gained two pounds this year, not huge but I already felt too heavy last year. The nurse said after menopause if you eat the same and exercise the same you'll gain at least two pounds every year; it's normal. You have to eat less or exercise more to maintain, and if you want to lose you have to work even harder. As you said, it's a lifestyle change. After awhile it becomes second nature and you don't even think about it.

"I've not eaten any crap this week on vacation, excluding three silly drinks by the pool, and I hope to keep it up at home. The hard one will be giving up the alcohol but I know I have to do it for awhile. A glass or two of wine at night is packing in the calories. My goal is to lose fifteen pounds and get more fit. Thanks for the motivation."

A FAT KID

Halyna said: "I was fat as a child and teenager, a total couch potato. I decided I didn't want to become like my mother, who was obese until I talked her into going on a diet and losing seventy pounds, but that's another story.

"When I was nineteen I started dieting and exercising and lost thirty pounds. Ultimately I lost another ten pounds. To do this and maintain my weight I wrote down everything I ate, including calories, at least five days per week for thirty years, stopping when I turned fifty. Now the calorie count of most of what I eat is ingrained into my brain. I've maintained the same weight for more than fifteen years."

BE SELFISH

John added: "I think the whole exercise and nutrition thing is that to do it well you have to be selfish — these two things have to be the top priority on your daily to-do list."

THERMODYNAMICS AND YOU

The First Law of Thermodynamics deals with the principle of conservation of energy. Energy can be changed from one form to another but it can't be created or destroyed.

The food we eat is converted into supplying energy for our bodies. If we consume 2,500 calories on a given day but only burn 2,000, the balance of 500 calories gets stored as fat for future use. Conversely, if we expend 3,000 calories in a given day by increasing our physical activity but continue to eat at the 2,500 level, we'll use up 500 of those stored fat calories.

A calorie is a calorie is a calorie. If you eat a healthy, low-fat dinner of fish, brown rice and salad with fat-free dressing, you can be proud of yourself. But, if over the course of the evening you precede the dinner with a gin and tonic plus two glasses of wine with dinner you've added about 500 "empty calories" to the menu. They don't have any redeeming energy value but they still count in the total. Are you better off with 200 calories of raw vegetables and hummus or 100 calories of a processed snack? You know the answer. If there's no nutrition, there's no value.

THE GOVERNMENT CAN HELP

The USDA website, myplate.gov, is an excellent source of information on balancing calories, what foods to eat, what to reduce and many other items. It's a book on a website, providing useful information for all audiences. It's written in clear language and is well worth a look.

FOOD TRUMPS PILLS

Many of us take a variety of vitamin supplements every day but the reality is that we can obtain all of the vitamins and minerals we need from eating a healthy diet. Pills are not absorbed as efficiently as vitamins in whole foods. However, many older adults will benefit from supplements providing B-12, vitamin D and calcium. If you're uncertain, check with your doctor.

BETSY'S STORY

In 2008, Betsy, then seventy, decided she wanted to make a change. She'd never been into exercise but she went to our fitness center in SW Florida and told them she wanted to work with a trainer. She connected with Rita, who helped her develop a program. Betsy showed up four days a week. She also purchased an armband exercise system, Exerspy, from the fitness company dotFIT, that told her how many calories she was burning daily.

Betsy felt better and got stronger but she didn't lose weight. She thought she wouldn't have to watch what she ate and drank — exercise would do it for her. She knew a good deal about dieting; as she told me,

"This wasn't my first rodeo."

She realized her trainer's advice was on target and read a new book, *The Mayo Clinic Diet: Eat Well. Enjoy Life. Lose Weight*. She cut out alcohol, ate lots of fruits and vegetables, small amounts of protein and no "white stuff." This program started in July 2010.

She decided to continue exercising four days per week and eat healthy but she didn't weigh herself as she had on previous diets. After three weeks she got on the scale and found she'd lost fifteen pounds. Today, less than five months later, she has lost — get ready for this — a total of fifty pounds.

Betsy said, "That's how it happened — almost by accident and quickly. It was the astonishment of losing the first twenty-one pounds in a little over a month that held my interest. I knew the rest would be slow but with patience, perseverance and Rita's coaching I'm feeling pretty good now. My biggest challenge is not to be one of the nine out of ten who gain it back.

"This is about the combination of regular exercise, a sensible diet and portion control plus determination and discipline. I needed the luxury of being accountable to Rita who taught me that perspiration, also known as 'sweat' won't kill you."

The ones who don't gain it back are the ones who make a lifestyle change; they make exercise and healthy eating a permanent part of their lives.

ADVICE FROM A BRIT

Tom, in his fifties, was a co-worker and is now a friend for over twenty years. He offered this advice in an email from his home in London: "I agree, it's healthy eating, not dieting. What's worked for me is to eat carbohydrates at breakfast and not again during the day. It has two effects — one, to reduce the total amount of calories I eat, and two, to make me realize how you don't *need* to overeat — bread at lunch and dinner, crisps and potatoes are all nice to eat but fill you up unnecessarily.

"Another tip that works for me is to find four or five Golden Rules like that and not get worried about the small transgressions elsewhere. Mine are: No carbohydrates after breakfast. No potato crisps (a talisman for me as I think they are the ultimate lazy food). Exercise three times a week. No desserts — this is easy for me as I never really liked them. Always get five servings a day of vegetables.

"I also substitute foods. I know I'm going to have to eat *something*, so I might as well eat what won't do me any harm. So, if before dinner I would have had hummus and crackers, I now have hummus and carrot sticks. It's a small difference but you can maintain a similar eating/social routine *and* make positive changes. I found daunting (and therefore didn't do it) the idea of eating *nothing* before supper or having no nibbles at a drinks party.

"I think older people might like that approach because many of them will have gotten themselves into a routine over thirty or forty years. An example is the drink before dinner — it's more a signal of the end to the day than the need to have a slug of alcohol. So, for three times a week, keep the routine of the pre-dinner drink but substitute only tonic versus gin or vodka and tonic or Virgin Mary for Bloody Mary. Add up the amount of alcohol and calories you don't take in over three months and small steps become big moves. That's why my emphasis on three-month time periods."

VICKI AND HEALTHY EATING

Vicki read a draft of this chapter and wrote: "It's a great summary of healthy eating. I was looking to be sure that you included 'the whites' and alcohol in the foods to watch. I eliminated 'whites' about three years ago to get control of hypoglycemic-type symptoms (my doctor told me there are very few true hypoglycemics). I'm no saint — I'll eat wedding cake and the bread before dinner at restaurants, but as a daily choice I read labels carefully and choose whole grains (wheat flour does not mean 100% whole grain!) and fruit, agave and occasionally pure honey for sweets. Don't be fooled by the label 'organic' — as you know, it can still be processed.

"Empty calories aside, alcohol also reduces our inhibitions, increasing the likelihood that we'll overeat when tempted. When I eliminated alcohol I dropped five pounds without consciously doing anything else differently. Two years later, when I dropped the whites, I went down another dress size, without consciously making any other diet changes. I'm now an easy size four, where I was encroaching on a size eight five years ago.

"Also — thanks to your nudge and my willingness to not let the fear of failure control me, I registered for my first mini-triathlon next month. I've been actively training for the swim/bike/run, and am now excited to go for it!"

LET'S REVIEW

- Knowing your cholesterol numbers is an important step in healthy living.
- Understanding the different types of fats is equally critical.
- Writing down what you eat and drink is a really big deal. The chances are very good that you'll eat less if you do this.
- Recent studies suggest that fiber intake, particularly from whole grains, is a big part of living a longer, healthy life.
- Drink water when you feel like it, but manage your intake of salt and be sure you're getting enough potassium.
- Too much sugar intake has become a national pastime. This is one to avoid.
- Processed food is not all bad; understand the differences.
- We regularly see articles talking about "a serving." It's important to know that all servings aren't created equal.

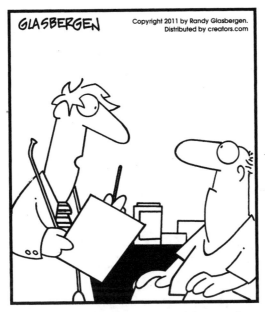

"**Spend more time outdoors with your dog.**
Teach him how to throw a stick
for you to chase."

CHAPTER ELEVEN — THE NEXT LEVEL

In the December 2010 issue of Men's Journal *Richard Branson, sixty, founder of Virgin Group, was asked, "How should a man handle getting older?" He said: "The absolute key to enjoying life, whether you're old or young, is looking after your body."*

HERE'S WHAT'S COMING

- We'll cover some advanced exercises that may appeal to you now or later.
- Let's talk a bit more about why to use a trainer.
- Here are some serious intervals that could be great for you.
- How much strength training should you do, in sets and reps?
- Time to revisit concentric and eccentric and why they matter.

What's prompted me to write this chapter is that a number of the reviewers of the manuscript who've made the most change in their exercise program were those who were already doing lots of exercise. The changes they made tended to be to add harder exercise, like serious interval training, and doing strength training to fatigue.

Participants in virtually all sports activities can be divided into those who are competitive, committed or recreational. I don't expect many readers to be competitive in the fitness category, although they may be in another sport such as golf or tennis. This chapter is directed at those who are committed to fitness, maybe primarily as a vehicle for maintaining their abilities in other activities.

This chapter includes some topics covered in the aerobics and strength training chapters but at a higher level. All interval training isn't the same, for example. We'll talk about the techniques and benefits of higher levels of intensity.

NEWTON'S FIRST LAW OF MOTION

"Every object in a state of uniform motion tends to remain in that state of motion unless an external force is applied to it." A reasonable question is "What does this have to do with advanced exercise?" Let me explain.

Based on my personal observation of a number of individuals — particularly men — who exercise a lot, I think they (including yours truly) tend to err on two fundamental issues:

- We get comfortable doing a series of exercises and stick with them way too long. They're like an old shoe to us. Why buy a new pair and go through the discomfort when the old pair feels so good? We'll continue in motion with our program unless we apply the external force of developing new exercises.

- We believe that we know as much, and maybe more, than any trainer, so why would we need to seek any advice on what we should do? We don't know what we don't know.

Cathy, the director of our fitness center in SW Florida, said, "To stick with an exercise program it's best to change your program every three weeks and not make it a chore by staying in the gym for two hours. You should be able to get everything done in fifty minutes, unless part of the purpose is to be social."

So what's the big deal, you say? Our bodies get used to doing the same thing over and over. Our muscles and our brain go on autopilot and receive minimal benefit from the process. New exercises add stress to muscle fibers and help develop new neuromuscular pathways.

Some people could make an argument, "I've been working out doing the same thing for fifteen years, I'm reasonably fit and strong and I don't get injured easily. Why should I change, I don't feel the need to be stronger."

The problem is that we lose muscle mass as we age. This process is called "sarcopenia," which is discussed in Chapter Seven. The best way to limit that loss is by varying strength training exercises and doing them to fatigue. No steroids, please.

WHAT ABOUT TRAINERS?

George said it well: "I've been using a personal trainer twice a week for the past two months after twenty-five years of not using one. The reason is that after reading your book, I became convinced that I wanted to invest in my future health." George is in excellent physical condition and has been exercising for decades. He recognized that he didn't know it all and could make significant improvement by learning from a professional.

The advice of health and fitness professionals is to hire a trainer. Give up some of your cherished exercises and "trick" your body by doing new exercises. If you don't connect with your first trainer, try another.

If you don't belong to a gym, do your exercises at home, or just don't want to go to the trouble of finding and hiring a trainer, then buy a few books that provide words and pictures of a variety of exercises and force yourself to do some new exercises. I'll list several good books at the end of this book.

MORE ABOUT INTERVALS

Two types of interval training have gained wide acceptance for serious athletes and even for those not so serious. They are physically demanding and are not designed for those new to endurance exercise. They can be done on treadmills, elliptical trainers, indoor or outdoor bikes, while running outdoors, swimming or brisk walking.

High Intensity Interval Training — These are periods of one to two minutes of high intensity —eighty percent to ninety percent of maximum heart rate (MHR) — followed by four minutes of normal activity in the sixty percent to seventy percent of MHR. Repeat the process two to four times.

Sprint Interval Training — These are short periods of thirty seconds of high intensity followed by cool down to sixty percent to seventy percent of MHR and then repeat the process. A good way to do this is to begin with an effort at sixty percent of MHR, cool down for two minutes, then do one at eighty percent of MHR, cool down for two minutes and then do several more at maximum intensity, followed by two to four minutes of recovery for each, depending on your conditioning.

VIEWS OF A PHYSICAL THERAPIST

David Ostrow, PT, is president of Body Balance for Performance, an organization with locations across the country focused on fitness training for golfers. David reviewed my manuscript as it was being written. Here's what he said about interval training:

"There's a HUGE body of science on the effects of interval training for caloric consumption, control of lipids and cardiac health. The science on this over the last ten years has grown exponentially.

"The parameters in the current research that I've seen suggest two types of interval training: high-intensity interval training (HIIT) and sprint interval training (SIT) training. The regimens for these are quite structured and produce better results on the cardiovascular system than lower level aerobic training as well as superior lipid control (LDL, HDL and triglycerides) than aerobic training, and SIT is much more effective than HIIT at this.

"The really interesting thing is that the science seems to indicate that there are diminishing returns after ten minutes of this training. Ten minutes in this mode creates higher metabolic rates and dramatic improvements over thirty to forty minutes of "aerobic" work at sixty percent to seventy percent of MHR. Stunning to me, but well documented — ten minutes of HIIT burns more calories, controls lipid profiles better and affects VO_2 max better than thirty minutes of aerobics at sixty percent to seventy percent of MHR.

"SIT is even more fascinating. The science there says one minute of SIT is even better than the HIIT approach for the same metrics. That's not to say it's a one-minute sprint, rather the accumulation of sixty seconds of sprint level activities over fifteen to twenty-five minutes. The science again says that more than a minute has diminishing returns so I discourage more than sixty seconds. This method involves extremely high-intensity activity "sprints" for ten to fifteen seconds with a three- to four-minute cool down between each sprint.

"During the cool down, body weight strength training or stretching or functional movement exercises are done at the low intensity interval. So sprint all out . . . feel like you're gonna puke at the end of the ten seconds. Consider this: the world's fastest man covers 100 meters in less than ten seconds. Most of us geezers will go half that distance in ten seconds and collapse just like the fastest in the world.

"If you choose ten seconds, which is my counsel to the population you're targeting, then do six ten-second intervals with three to four minutes of other activity . . . that's a total of twenty-five minutes during which you get strength, functional and mobility work — the complete workout — for the senior. Remember the scientific data on SIT show that it's better than HIIT.

"Both protocols say every other day is most effective. That means on a two-week cycle — Monday, Wednesday, Friday, Sunday, Tuesday, Thursday, Saturday, repeat. The science is clear on the need for 36–48 hours of recovery for maximum effectiveness.

"What I don't know is if these modes of training are in tune with aerobics effects on brain function — that would be an interesting study.

"Does this sound too hard for geezers? These are what most of our clients are doing now. Remember you are my demographic . . . the target of your book is too. The beauty of both of these modes is that they can be done on any piece of equipment, including swimming, streets, grass, sidewalks, treadmills, bikes, elliptical trainers — anything. It's the timing and intensity that matter, according to the science."

A study at McMaster University led by doctoral student Mark Rakabowchuk supports what David Ostrow says on the previous two pages. The study compared individuals doing interval training for thirty-second all-out sprints three times a week to a group that completed moderate-intensity cycling forty to sixty minutes, five days a week. They found that the shorter-term, high-intensity exercise produced similar results.

They also found that six weeks of sprint interval training was as effective at improving the structure and function of arteries as longer endurance exercises requiring more time commitment.

INTERVAL SUMMARY

Intervals are really a big deal for a variety of reasons:

- You can accomplish more in less time, important to many. In the process you can improve both aerobic and anaerobic fitness. Endurance training at a lower level of intensity focuses on aerobic fitness only.

- Intervals improve vascular health and decrease the risk of cardiovascular disease.

- You can get faster and stronger in a shorter period of time. Walkers who are comfortable walking three and a half miles per hour may find four miles an hour very manageable. Cyclists frequently find that their average speed increases by ten percent or more.

- Remember the discussion of fast-twitch and slow-twitch muscles? Interval training activates the fast-twitch muscle fibers, the ones we have to work the most to keep as we age.

MIRKIN ON ENDURANCE

Gabe Mirkin published an article on his website recently, "Intense Training Maintains Endurance in Older People." He told the story of himself and his wife, seventy-five and sixty-nine, respectively, competing in a bike tandem event in Sebring, FL. They covered the fifty-one miles at an average speed of nineteen miles per hour.

Gabe said, "You lose power and strength with aging, but you keep most of your endurance. If you train intensely, you can maintain the size and number of mitochondria in muscles that use oxygen to convert food to energy, which helps you keep your ability to move faster over long distances."

STRENGTH TRAINING

Chapter Six on strength training provides a good base for this topic, but let's discuss a few issues in a bit more detail. Remember a fundamental principle of strength training — if there is no overload on muscles, there's no improvement in strength. We need to lift weights to fatigue in order to increase our strength.

Suppose you're sixty-eight years old and have done strength training regularly for ten years, though not to fatigue. You've done two sets of medium-level weights for fifteen repetitions each time, but at the end of the last set you're far from fatigued. You can easily do another five repetitions each time, maybe even more, but don't. What'll happen if you started lifting heavier weights for eight to twelve repetitions each time, maybe increasing to three sets, adding more weight to the third set so that the best you can do is eight to ten repetitions?

The answer is that you'll generate hypertrophy, which is muscle enlargement. You'll break down the muscle fibers — cells — and they'll grow back stronger. You can recover some of the muscle mass you've lost over the years. You'll activate muscle fibers that you're not calling on when you're working at a more moderate level of intensity.

What about free weights versus machines? The research tends to support free weights as the better choice. Free weights can provide greater specificity of training as well as movement versatility, plus they require both balance and stability beyond that needed with machines. As we age, balance and coordination become even more critical. Firing those nerve fibers during exercise is the process of proprioception.

There are exercises that don't use weights that are terrific for building strength. Examples are push-ups, chin-ups and dips.

HOW MUCH IS ENOUGH?

How many sets and how many repetitions is a very good question. The answer is, "It depends." Highly trained athletes require four to eight sets per muscle group of varying number of repetitions to achieve maximum strength gains. Those reading this book don't fall into that category.

For the readers of this book two to three sets will provide the level of intensity needed to achieve muscle gain or maintenance. As far as the number of repetitions, those working to fatigue may find that they can do ten to twelve repetitions for the first set but perhaps only eight to ten for the second or third set.

HOW MANY REPETITIONS?

Roger, a kinesiologist, said, "I was working out the other day, doing some upper body work on one of the machines in the fitness center and got to thinking about working to fatigue and building muscles.

"As you know there are two principles: low repetitions, high resistance to build strength, and low resistance, high repetitions for endurance. It just didn't make sense that it was either/or. When I do ten to twelve reps, but work to fatigue, it's doing both, and not making the strain on my muscles too great. For me, once I get to twelve reps, I increase the resistance, can do eight to ten at the new resistance and work at that level for awhile. I am still going to fatigue, yet not overdoing it.

"I asked the head of the Fitness Centre about it, and he said I was correct. The key is to produce to fatigue and ultimately to gradually increase resistance so that muscles have to work harder as they get stronger. This is something to consider for older adults, rather than doing the maximum four to six reps to fatigue, as really well-conditioned weight lifters do.

"Hope all is going well. Spring has finally arrived here. I went for my first run outdoors since last October; felt good, though I might have overdone it a bit, as feeling quite stiff now. Some good wine should help that."

VARIETY HELPS

Consider varying your exercise program by doing ascending and descending ladders. You do ascending by beginning with a lighter weight that you know you can do fifteen times and then add weight to the level you can do only ten to twelve times. For the third set add more weight so that you can only do eight to ten reps. The next gym day reverse the process and begin with the heaviest weight and work down to the lighter one.

CONCENTRIC AND ECCENTRIC

It sounds counterintuitive, but lowering a weight slowly versus quickly produces more muscle gain than the act of raising it. If you take two seconds to raise dumbbells, take four or more to lower them. Raising the weight shortens the muscle length while lowering it increases the muscle length. It's likely not possible to lower the weight too slowly. Muscles, as they lengthen, are able to produce more force, so as you slowly lower the weight — in a position where it's not possible to shorten the muscle because of fatigue — strengthening is occurring.

LEN'S STORY

"I'm a sixty-eight-year-old guy active in kayaking, bicycling and jogging but haven't done any serious upper body exercise for many years due to a problem in my right arm. I had a recurring problem with pain in my right shoulder and upper arm that was diagnosed as arthritis. The worst part was that it occasionally kept me from my passion, kayaking.

"My paddling buddy Art suggested I consider joining a gym and then pointed me to Harry's book. After a few hours of reading I got inspired and started following the suggestions he outlined. I hired a trainer, a seventy-three-year-old incredibly conditioned guy who specializes in senior training, to get me started.

"I got into a routine of at least an hour in the early morning three days a week, doing a complete circuit of the weight training machines followed by a series of exercises with dumbbells. On off days I sometimes do a series of exercises using the large exercise ball. At the start I was favoring the right arm/shoulder and using lower right side weights with the dumbbells. After a few weeks I was shocked as the pain in the right arm/shoulder began to clear up and I progressed to higher weights.

"Now, after almost three months, I have no soreness in the right arm/shoulder and can do all sorts of kayak rolls and paddle for hours with no pain at all. The exercising has built up the muscles around the affected area enough to give sufficient support to eliminate the pain.

"I was paddling casually with Art and two other friends a few days ago and we had a little over a mile to go to the take-out site. I said that I'd go ahead and take out my boat first so I could help the others. I started paddling at a faster pace and soon fell into a nice rhythm that I knew was faster than normal for our casual trips.

"When I reached the shore I looked back and Art was quite a bit ahead of the other guys and behind me. Art has always been a faster paddler than I as he is a serious "gym rat" and has developed a strong upper body. He shocked me when he said that he was having trouble keeping up with me — something that had never happened before.

"So, as a sixty-eight-year-old would-be athlete I finally got back into a regular strength training program as outlined in Harry's book and am extremely pleased with the substantial progress I've made in a few short months. Other areas in Harry's book have also been very helpful as I have an implanted pacemaker (only in back-up mode, not pacing me) and a few years ago had my mitral valve replaced along with a triple bypass, so I'm determined to keep very active. My goal is to maintain and build upon this strength-training program along with my jogging and bicycling — for the rest of my life."

SPECIAL EXERCISE PROGRAMS

There are several exercise programs available at either specific locations, online or via DVDs that provide a great deal of variety as well as, in some cases, the advantage of working with a support group. The ones I've read about and had some friends participate in are Crossfit, Boot Camp and P90X. You can Google any one of these and find out whether there's a location near you. I believe P90X is only available as DVDs.

LET'S REVIEW

- It's nice to have some favorite exercises, but don't get married to them. Change your program on a regular basis so that your body will learn new routines.

- Utilizing a personal trainer on a regular basis is an excellent investment.

- Intervals are a powerful way to get more out of your time invested, plus help your heart.

- When you're doing strength training, remember the power of concentric and eccentric to get more out of your workout.

CHAPTER TWELVE — EPILOGUE: THE FUTURE BELONGS TO THE FIT

"The future depends on what we do in the present." — Mahatma Gandhi, 1869–1948

SUCCESS

"Success is the peace of mind which is a direct result of self-satisfaction in knowing you made the *effort* to become the best you are capable of becoming." — John Wooden, 1910–2010

There's a small evolution going on in this country. More and more individuals, particularly those in their fifties and beyond, are becoming aware of their remaining time on this earth. They're realizing that both the length and the quality of their years are dependent on what they do — now — to take care of themselves. Many would like to live a longer, healthier life and are willing to do the things that will help make that happen.

NOW'S THE TIME

You've now read a book of several hundred pages written by a man who has a passion for fitness and health. I've observed the positive effects of exercise and healthy eating, both personally and with a number of my friends and family. I've also, unfortunately, seen those who are unwilling or unable to change their life.

If you were already active in fitness and healthy eating prior to reading this book, I hope that it's motivated you to do even more. This has happened with a number of my friends who devoted many hours to critiquing my manuscript during its development. Their positive feedback in the early stages provided motivation for me to stay the course.

If you're not already active in fitness and healthy eating, I hope you'll decide that now's the time. "Sooner trumps later," "The early bird catches the worm" and all of those other quotations we used to hear as kids, including "The longer you wait, the harder it is to both get going and keep going." Maybe I just invented the last one, I don't know for sure.

AGE ISN'T A BARRIER

Pat, in her early fifties, said: "I'm on vacation for a week in Colorado and the skiing has been amazing. I'm so much stronger and have more stamina so I enjoy my favorite sport even more. But what really inspires me is talking with the much older people I've met on chairlifts who are fit, energetic and raring to go. I sat with one person who's seventy-five and skis all the time with his wife, also seventy-five. Two other guys, also in their seventies, were great skiers, too. Age isn't a barrier; attitude and physical state can be, but we have control over those.

"The best news yet is that my husband Jon is now totally into fitness. He's lost thirty pounds and is skiing harder and better than ever. He looks great and has much more energy. Being in Colorado has made a difference for him because there is a culture of fitness here in the mountains. Exercise, eat right, find things you love to do and the future is bright. The future really does belong to the fit."

THE GOOD NEWS AND BAD NEWS ABOUT CHANGE

The classic question: Which do you want first, the good news or the bad news? Let's begin with the good news.

The good news is that we're capable of both neurogenesis — the growth of new brain cells — and neuroplasticity — the ability to learn new information and get our brains to remember it — even at an advanced age. Our brains create synapses, or connections, that remember new activities; the more we do them, the stronger the connections. This process is called synaptic plasticity. A man or woman in their seventies can learn new skills; we're not out to pasture just yet.

The bad news is that if we haven't been doing activities that stretch our brains on a regular basis — taking on some we've never done before — it takes more time and energy to succeed. What a teenager could master in hours can take older adults days. That can be downright discouraging.

Many of you have heard the question, "How do you get really good at golf?" The answer is, "Begin at an earlier age."Men and women who start playing golf in their fifties or sixties can find it immensely frustrating. Their brains have to work hard to adapt to the demands of a sport that's somewhat unique in its mental and physical requirements. It takes lots of practice to reach even an average level of proficiency.

The same holds true for developing and maintaining motivation to improve fitness and healthy eating. Keeping at a program that has new physical and mental requirements isn't easy. It's much easier to quit than keep at it. We can all rationalize why we can either put off starting a program "until a better time," or quit when we've started because "we're just too busy." Most of us have had lots of practice developing those rationalization skills. Those synapses are well-developed.

Nike says, "Just do it"; Alcoholics Anonymous says, "Fake it until you make it"; Chip and Dan Heath say in their book, *Switch: How to Change Things When Change is Hard,* to find an Action Trigger — something that will follow or precede your commitment and action. They also say, "When you set small, visible goals, and people achieve them, they start to get into their heads that they can succeed."

Neale added: "One of the undercurrents in the book is about how to make big changes in your life: make lots of little changes consistently over time and, voila, you've made a big change."

Numerous research studies have shown that being part of a support group can be a game changer. Not only are you no longer trying to do something solo but you have others who are providing encouragement as well as expecting the same from you. A support group, even if it's only two people, can be the difference between success and failure. They can even be long distance, updating and encouraging each other by phone or email.

COGNITIVE DISSONANCE

Some readers might be experiencing cognitive dissonance. This is an important theory of social psychology that describes how we can hold conflicting ideas simultaneously. You may have believed that the steps you've been taking to manage your health and fitness were sufficient, only to read a book that says otherwise. You now may have conflicting beliefs.

One reviewer informed me that he eats two meals a day and weighs the same as he did ten years ago. He also said that the food he eats bears no relationship to the recommendations in this book. He does a modest amount of exercise and doesn't plan to increase it. His rationale is that he has good genes; his parents lived into their nineties, he's never been in a hospital (not even for his birth) and he feels fine.

This view ignores the fact that he has lost and will continue to lose muscle mass while increasing the percentage of visceral fat in his body. While he may well live into his nineties due to his genes, the quality of his life will likely, at some point, be impacted by his limited exercise and lack of healthy eating. He's suspended belief in the value of making changes in his behavior.

The same can be true for someone who smokes, knowing full well the effect it can have on their health. They might say, "I'm going to die of something, so it might as well be from smoking." I don't think we need to analyze the fallacy in this thinking.

Many of the reviewers of this book have said that reading it has motivated them to rethink the exercise they do as well as what they eat and drink. They've learned that what they were doing isn't enough and that they can increase the odds of living a longer, active, healthier life by making some changes. Whether you make a similar decision is, of course, totally up to you.

My wife Deb has lunch with friends regularly at a restaurant nearby. Several times her server was Andy, an energetic, enthusiastic woman. Deb learned that she's also a personal trainer. The statement on her card is "Live Fit — There Is No Finish Line." What a great summary.

PERFECTION

Vince Lombardi said, "Perfection is not attainable, but if we chase perfection we can catch excellence." Let's face it, we're not going to show up for exercise every day or we're going to eat the wrong foods sometimes. On those days we won't achieve either perfection or excellence. The key is to get over it, get back on track and congratulate ourselves for what we do achieve. We can have lots of excellent days.

WILLPOWER

Willpower: Rediscovering the Greatest Human Strength by Baumeister and Tierney was published in 2011. I found the content very relevant.

One of their ideas: "The best way to reduce stress in your life is to stop screwing up. That means setting up your life so that you have a realistic chance to succeed." Can you think of anything more relevant to exercise and healthy eating?

They say that our supply of willpower is freshened every day, but the total for the day is limited. Maybe that's why those who exercise early in the day likely have more success at sticking with the program. Later in the day we've depleted our day's supply of willpower on other things.

A few of their other ideas:

Pick Your Battles — Focus on doing the things that are most important in your life, the ones that will make the most difference over the long run. This isn't a daily exercise but perhaps a monthly one, a time to review what progress you've made on priorities and where you should focus your energy going forward. Don't expect perfection; the goal should be to show improvement over time.

Keep Track — "Monitoring is crucial for any kind of plan you make — and it can even work if you don't make a plan at all. Weighing yourself every day or keeping a food diary can help you lose weight, just as tracking your purchases will help you spend less." They also mention that just knowing that you've got to record information will discourage procrastination, and the better job you do of monitoring, the greater chance of success.

A big advantage of keeping track is that you can go back and review your accomplishments if you have a period when you don't complete your goals, show up for exercise, eat healthy, whatever. It's a reminder that you are capable of getting back on the right track.

Reward Often — We all need some reward for achieving goals we've set. If we set a goal of losing twenty pounds, we should determine a suitable reward for doing it. Maybe it's dinner at a very nice restaurant, or how about a new pair of pants and a new belt?

One last quote: "Self-control is ultimately about much more than self-help. It's essential for savoring your time on earth and sharing joy with the people you love."

TWO OLD GUYS AT THE GYM

Art passed on this story about a session at his gym in Sarasota, FL: "I met a couple of interesting guys at the gym this afternoon. As I walked into the corner of the gym where they have the core equipment set up there was an old timer adding weights to his friend's exercise bar without his friend's knowledge. Eventually he figured it out and we were all laughing. I started talking to the 'weight adder,' Joel. He grew up in Newton, MA, earned his Ph.D. in political science at Columbia University and taught for his entire career at New York University, Washington Square.

"About forty years ago he had back problems; he started swimming and swam for twenty years without back problems. He moved to Sarasota and decided he never wanted to see the bottom of another pool. He started going to the gym and is now in his twentieth year of gym exercise. He's eighty-seven years old, has never been seriously ill and is happily married.

"I then started talking to another old guy, Tom. He asked me to guess how old he was. I played it safe, thought he was in his late eighties also so I guessed eighty-four; he's ninety-four. A native of Brooklyn, NY, he served in Germany in WWII. He started running in his sixties and ran the New York Marathon at age sixty-six, finishing in 4:09. He's still married to his first wife.

"Years ago he was a heavy smoker, coughed a lot and went to a doctor for X-rays. The doctor gave him three years to live. Tom quit smoking and quit his job as a jeweler, went to school on the GI bill, became a nutritionist and worked for a variety of public institutions in New York until he retired. He works out almost every day and gets plenty of rest also.

"Both of these guys attributed their vitality to their exercise programs."

THE MAGIC OF THINKING BIG

David Schwartz wrote a book with this title in the late 1950s; it's sold over four million copies and continues to sell well today. David was one of my professors at Georgia State University in Atlanta and we became good friends. I've met people over the years who've told me that reading David's book changed their lives. The message of the book is to think bigger about how to achieve success and happiness.

I thought of this book after a dinner recently with Mark. I mentioned to him that I'd just realized that if this book is successful and motivates a number of individuals to improve their fitness and healthy eating, it will be one of the most important things I've ever done, right behind raising a son who's turned out to be a very fine human being. Mark suggested I mention this in the book. I'll have done this at age seventy-three, a time when we're theoretically "over the hill." I hope reading it has a positive impact on your life and that it's made you think bigger about your fitness and health.

What can you do that would add more meaning to your life and that of others? Maybe it's to take care of yourself so that you can lead a longer, active, healthy life, plus be a positive force and role model for your children and grandchildren. Maybe you have a set of talents that can benefit others. Who knows, maybe you might even write a book.

WHAT REVIEWERS HAVE DONE

Following are some of the stories I've collected during the process of writing this book. They're written by people who were kind enough to read my material in manuscript form and, in many cases, offer advice on how to make it better. The stories are comments they made along the way about what they've done as a result of reading the manuscript.

I've gotten a lot of satisfaction out of seeing that so many of my reviewers have taken the message to heart and improved their own exercise and eating habits. After all, this is exactly why I wrote the book. This provides encouragement to think that a significant number of readers of the final, published book may take similar action. I hope these stories can provide motivation to others.

NOTES FROM A SMALL ISLAND

Tom is a native of England, has a home near Oxford. These are his comments following reviewing my first ten chapters:

"I haven't even bought your book and am getting fitter by the day! I set a series of goals at the New Year's to conclude before Easter (3.75 months) which, generally, have had a good effect:

- To give up drink — one or two lapses — but I haven't missed it much (that's worrying in itself).

- To lose weight — I was 208 pounds on January 1 and am now down to 198 pounds with my aim to be at 194 by Easter. I think I'll get to 196 but not sure of the last two pounds, but 196 will take me back to a weight last seen in 1999.

- To exercise more — I dusted off the Concept rowing machine and set about a series of different distances. The main comparative one is 5,000 meters. This morning I got to a recent low of eighteen minutes, thirty-one seconds. That compares to eighteen minutes, ten seconds when I last did it competitively in 2003, so I'm very happy with the progress. I've only had one spin on my bike this year — eighteen miles last weekend — which was fun.

"Looking back at where I was in January in my times and indicators on the rowing machine, I can see a real fall in times that accelerated in the last six weeks — keep at it, keep the long-term view. You mention it in the habit-changing chapter, but it takes three months to develop a habit I'm sure.

"I found a buddy — my brother-in-law is doing the same weight loss and exercise regimen. We call each other on Saturday mornings. It's a huge motivator to share and compete.

"I like the 'substitution' concept as a motivator too — substituting exercise for something I used to do by car or lift — and keeping a note of that. Example: I have to go to the shops each day but I substituted walking for the car three times this week. I have to go to the office each day but I substituted the stairs three times instead of the lift — it helps people think that they don't have to do MORE to exercise — they simply replace.

"I know the BHAG story but I think you need to emphasise that measuring/setting goals on a wider range of indicators is good — am I still out of breath when I climb the stairs? How many days in a week did I not drink alcohol? How often did I walk to the shops rather than drive?"

HE LOVES FIT AND SORE

Russ wrote the following after we met in the spring of 2011. He had heard me talking about my book and asked if I would send him a copy of the manuscript:

"Harry, thanks for the advance copy of your book. I'm loving it. I just turned fifty-five on Sunday. I've been a gym rat since about ninth grade, so you're truly preaching to the choir. My Dad lived until eighty-five and ran most days until his late seventies. My Mom died several years ago at ninety; she walked her 'Miracle Mile' most days in New Hampshire until her last year. I suppose that I come by my love of exercise genetically. My daughter is sixteen and likes to go the gym with me regularly, as long as I don't let on that we're related.

"Your book has reenergized me. I'm now focusing on the interval training aspect that you espouse. I've also started to log my workouts. Both of these measures are providing additional motivation for me. I work on taking one or two days a week off. If, for some unforeseen reason, I can't get my anticipated workout in, my skin feels like it wants to crawl off of my body. I guess I'm truly hooked. Your opus has helped me 'keep it fresh.'

"I'm enjoying my changing of workouts more than my previous few variations. I'm now stiff and/or sore more often and I LOVE that feeling. It reminds me of that feeling after high school basketball 'two a days.' I don't know if this will all lead to a longer life, but I'm certain that it's leading me to a happier one.

"The Nike Fit app is helping me in the 'keep it fresh department.' It's full of variations that I've never done, or ones I've forgotten. With my appreciation, Russ."

RIDING THE TOWPATH

Chris, a sports orthopedist, wrote this after reading the" Exercise and the Brain" chapter:

"I really liked this chapter. Enough anecdotes to get information across which was well done. Overall, this is the best chapter written so far. If anyone can read this chapter and not want to get out, they're crazy. Did I tell you I've started riding the towpath?

"I've been doing spin classes this winter. You've convinced me and I'm just proofing the book!"

THE CURMUDGEON

Art W, a friend for over forty years, was my very first critic. Somewhere in the process he wrote: "As you know, I too have been a lifelong fitness enthusiast. While my enthusiasms have shifted over the years depending on where I was living and the time I could make available to pursue my sport of the moment, I have to say that reading your manuscript has rejuvenated my resolve to keep moving.

"Eight months ago I was feeling pretty good about my activity level of exercising three or four days a week. Now I'm up to five or six days a week and feeling better for it. Sue notices the decrease in my curmudgeonly tendencies and offers (makes me go out and do it) a lot of support. Keep it up."

BACK WITH THE PROGRAM

David, a physical therapist, is president of a golf fitness company: "This is superb. Well done. I love the aerobics and brain function chapter, and strength-training section too. I have several comments that I hope you'll take constructively as that's the intention.

"I believe you're onto something here, Harry. Today I did my body weight strength training and HIIT training for the first time in years. I want the benefits and somehow you with this book have gotten to me in a way that no one else has . . . Thank you."

WALKING AGAIN

Ruth, who's not been into regular exercise, wrote: "I like your style, conversational and upbeat. I also like meeting your friends in the book . . . a good personal touch.

"And maybe it isn't an accident that after starting your book I renewed my walking program (abandoned after a very long almost year-long PAINFUL bout with planter's fasciitis.) Just a couple of weeks of regular walking, over ten miles a week, and I'm more alert. 'Really?' says my husband. I've also started stretching exercises in the morning using a book, *Yoga for Seniors*."

HELPING A DRUG ADDICT

George, a very fit friend in SW Florida, wrote this after reading the first seven chapters:

"This book is a gem! It has real power. It can change lives. Not for an hour or a day or a week or a month, but for years — for the rest of one's life.

"I thought I knew a lot about aerobic fitness, the brain and motivation. After all, I've spent a large part of the past twenty-five years running, hiking, biking and working out in the gym, trying to stay young. Your book is helping me get to the next level.

"I have a confession to make. I've been sharing your book, a little at a time, with a young man, twenty years old, who's a drug addict. My hope is that he'll take some of your human-interest stories to heart as he struggles to get his life back on track.

"As a result of reading this I've been using a personal trainer twice a week after twenty-five years of not using one. I became convinced that I wanted to invest in my future health. I'll reassess my eating habits when I reread the appropriate chapters."

JOHN'S PRIORITIES

John lives in Newburyport, MA, a beautiful town on the Merrimac River, just as it enters the Atlantic Ocean. He said: "After reading your manuscript I changed my priorities of what's important in my life. Daily exercise now comes first. I have to force myself to take a day off every six to eight days. I do strength training more often and continue to ramp up my pace with intervals on the elliptical machine. At the supermarket I pay more attention to product label disclosures (fat, additives, and sugars). I'm anxious to see the book published so I can share it with friends and colleagues."

MAKING A DIFFERENCE

Mark, a friend in SW Florida, said: "Thanks for the opportunity to give some input, Harry. You asked me if I liked the book. Wrong question. Will it make a difference in the way I manage my life? Well, I'm glad you asked.

"The primary benefit for me so far has been motivational and educational. The clear explanations of exercise physiology in the manuscript combined with the practical, no-nonsense approach appeals to me.

"On Tuesday when you called I was out riding my bike (not interval training, mind you, but I was riding), and the following day I spent an hour and a half in the gym, including some intervals during my thirty minutes on the treadmill. Get the book finished soon so I can buy a copy and keep up the motivation. By the way, I did think that the chapter on the brain was a blockbuster and the highlight of a very enjoyable book.

"Thanks for letting me in on the process. I'm looking forward to a summer in the pool, strength training in the gym, walking the golf course in North Carolina and creating a more healthy diet. I might even begin to drink a little less — we can dream, can't we?"

LOOKING FOR BALANCE

David, a friend in Santa Barbara, CA, read the first eight chapters: "I just finished and must say it makes one think. You have a lot of very useful information in it and the individual stories are really great because they have more impact than a 'thou should' approach.

"I must say that it got me thinking about my life and attitude to working out. It seems that throughout I've always had an inner drive to do some kind of exercise, but not as structured or with the kind of focus as you recommend. The closest I came was when I felt 'rich' and had a personal trainer I worked out with three times a week. I also had a massage once a week — now that was fantastic.

"What I've been lacking is the kind of overall balance you talk about throughout the book. It's been on my mind for quite awhile.

"It's a good book that I'm sure will be wonderful when you've got it all together. Based on what I've read it would be one I'd recommend to everyone; and frankly, it will benefit younger folk. While there is a general increase in fitness books, there's nothing I'm aware of that is as specific or as broadly relevant as what you're creating.

"Your book has an important message and needs to be present for people to see it and hopefully absorb its message, so I wish you every success."

In 1987, David started and finished the RAAM (Race Across America), a 3,000-mile cycling race from San Francisco to the Washington Monument. Outside *magazine calls is "the toughest test of endurance in the world." (The race is now run from Oceanside, CA, to Annapolis, MD.) He said, "I was the penultimate official finisher, right behind Jim Pensyres. I refer to it as my 'temporary lapse of reason,' in homage to Pink Floyd."*

TAKING ACTION

Bob, from SW Florida, has never been into exercise. He read the first seven chapters of the manuscript and said: "Harry — I enjoyed reading the book more than I thought I would. It's well-paced and full of interesting, real stories. I found myself wanting to read on. I believe that you certainly make the case for 'proper exercise' if one wants to retain an active, robust quality of life late into one's years. I don't think the book is too technical, although those sections were of less interest to me. The technical aspects do add credibility. I'll be interested in the nutritional chapter when it's completed. I believe your objective is to move people to action, and you did that with me!"

LOTS OF CHANGES

Sandy and Ann live in upstate New York. I sent them the manuscript at the request of David from Santa Barbara, a mutual friend. They both wrote stories that are included earlier in the book.

"Harry, here's what we've changed as a result of reading your manuscript:

- We both now wear our heart monitors whenever we exercise and keep track of what fitness zone we're in, maximum heart rate, average rate, etc.

- We both added interval training into our bike workout, indoors on trainers for the winter.

- When weight lifting I bring back the weights much more slowly and with greater concentration than I did before reading your book.

- Overall, we always exercised and marked on the calendar what we did, but after reading your manuscript we schedule specific times into our day to work out.

- Nutrition-wise, we've added more fruits, lessened the salt and focused more on how much we put on our plates."

ENHANCED

Bill H in SW Florida has been a terrific reviewer throughout the process. He added: "In some respects I'm sorry that the book is almost finished but am sure you're very relieved. It's a great job, very motivational and truly a labor of love for you. I was pleased to be a small part of it and reading it has enhanced my life; maybe not changed, but definitely enhanced. You've done a wonderful job and a very good thing for many others. Congratulations!"

THE POWER OF WRITING IT DOWN

Vicki, a friend in SW Florida, is a terrific athlete. She periodically cycles with "The Big Boys" and has no trouble keeping up — she did a sixty-mile ride with us recently. This is the story of her first triathlon:

"I, a notorious workout junkie, found a number of sections in your book to be motivating and educational:

- The program of interval training to improve performance in aerobic activities.

- The research summarized in 'Exercise and the Brain.'

- The importance of a core exercise program, which a physical therapist designed for me.

- The importance of stretching, which your writing encouraged me to incorporate — for the first time in my life — into my fitness routine.

"You're preaching to the choir to convince me of the importance of incorporating exercise as part of our daily routine. But, from your book, I've gleaned that there's *exercise*, and there's *proper exercise with a plan and a goal*!

"This leads me to my personal experience, as a result of reading your manuscript. Over the years, I've been asked if I was training for a triathlon, probably because I mix up my aerobic routine — elliptical, bike, running, rowing, etc. My stock answer was always, 'No, I don't swim laps.'

"Two years ago, I decided to take swimming lessons, so I could add swimming to my aerobics. Was it hard! I couldn't even make it one lap across the pool, but I stayed the course and reached my goal. Now I could think about trying a triathlon.

"I found I couldn't commit to registering — fear of failure is a powerful deterrent to motivation. In your book you suggested that I write down my goal: 'I will register for and participate in a triathlon.' I finally wrote that letter of intent to you and last weekend completed my first triathlon at the age of fifty-six. I was far from the youngest person competing, but I can say without a doubt that I believe I was the happiest.

"What did I learn? Write down your goal, work toward it and accomplish it with great satisfaction! Thank you, Harry!"

A HYPOTHETICAL BIRTHDAY CELEBRATION

Following is a story of what I'd like to have happen when I turn ninety in seventeen years:

"For my ninetieth birthday I took my family on a cycling and sightseeing trip to Italy, one of our favorite countries. My son Michael and his wife Michelle brought along a tandem that can be taken apart and packed into two suitcases. I shipped my bike over as did my grandson (Harry Jr., of course) — a carbon fiber bike I'd gotten him for his last birthday. My wife Deb was along for the celebration and sightseeing.

"We'd done almost fifty miles that day and were headed up the last mountain to our hotel at the top. Harry Jr., fifteen years old, was in the lead, naturally. I was right behind him, Michael and Michelle bringing up the rear. It was a long climb with a fairly steady six-degree elevation. We were all working hard.

"A few hundred yards before the summit, where Deb was waiting with her camera, Michael got feisty and passed me; I tucked in behind him. Then, about fifty yards from the summit, I got a burst of adrenalin and slowly eased by Michael and Michelle. I beat them to the top by the length of a tire. Harry Jr. was way ahead of us.

"Deb took a great picture of the duel and then one of all of us together, tired and happy. We cleaned up and celebrated with a nice bottle of Barolo wine."

Early in the book I mentioned that we started a new program at our Florida fitness center called "Living a Healthy Life." The goal is to have members view the fitness center as a place to change and enhance the quality of their life, not just get some exercise. Part of the process is to set a BIG goal that can provide real motivation for the long term. Jim Collins calls them BHAG — Big Hairy Audacious Goals.

I mentioned my BHAG: "*I want to do what I do today seventeen years from now.*" That means that I want to do eighty at eighty and ninety at ninety — cycling miles on one ride, not golf score. Every year since I turned seventy we do a birthday ride in Bucks County, PA — my son and several close friends — and the minimum ride is my age. I want to do it when I'm ninety and Italy would be a wonderful place to celebrate.

If I really want my BHAG to happen, that means I have to think about what I do today that can impact what I'll be able to do in future years. Remember "The Butterfly Effect" in Chapter Nine? What I eat and drink today, and the exercise I do, will determine whether I can meet that BHAG.

Part of my motivation is to think about ideas like this imaginary birthday trip to Italy with my family, one of whom hasn't even been born yet. If I dream big, maybe I can do it.

I hope you have some big dreams and make them happen.

WHAT HAVE I LEARNED?

The way I remember it is "If you really want to learn something, be assigned to teach it." I'd add, "Or write about it." The person who's benefitted the most from this book is me, the guy who wrote it.

I've learned an enormous amount about every topic — motivation, exercise and the brain, aerobics, strength training, healthy eating, you name it — addressed in this book. Some of the learning contradicted what I thought I knew, leading to cognitive dissonance. That's a good thing; I had to change my thinking based on new information on several occasions.

Have I made a dramatic change in my lifestyle? I definitely eat differently: no fried food, much less red meat, lots of chicken and fish. I already ate lots of fruits and vegetables. I now know how much I eat daily and how much exercise I need to do to maintain my weight. The good news is that I enjoy the exercise — most days. If I'm not in the mood I do it anyway.

I now work harder when I do strength training, doing more exercises to fatigue. I'm stretching more, something I'd gotten out of the habit of doing regularly. A good trainer corrected that problem.

I do many more intervals while cycling. I now understand the value of intervals to both maintain and increase my athletic ability in my septuagenarian years and beyond. Not long ago one of my strongest cycling buddies followed me up an overpass — what counts as a hill in SW Florida — and said, "You couldn't go up that fast a year ago." He was right.

Recently I beat an athletic man at least thirty years my junior up the same overpass; he was amazed — as was I. He suggested we do another but I declined, knowing full well what the outcome would be. I learned long ago: "Don't push your luck." A more appropriate quote is from Clint Eastwood: "A man's got to know his limitations."

How does it feel to be seventy-three and able to do many of the things I did fifteen or twenty years ago? Frankly, absolutely fantastic. I hope you'll choose to join me.

YOUR KEYS TO SUCCESS IN FITNESS

Based upon the significant amount of research available as well as the comments from my team of over fifty reviewers, following is my summary of the keys to success.

Write It Down — The power of the written word for short-term and long-term goals, as well as recording exercise activity and eating habits, is significant. We're much more likely to take action when we write things down. It also helps to share our goals with others.

Variety — Remember Einstein's definition of insanity; "Doing the same thing over and over again and expecting different results." We need to modify our exercise routine frequently to obtain the best results. It's okay to keep a few favorites, but the body needs change.

Support — The research shows that those who are part of a support group, even if it's only a group of two, are much more likely to stay the course. The support can even be long distance communication and encouragement via email and telephone.

Intervals — They're powerful. We get stronger and faster when we do interval training, whether it's walking, running, cycling or using gym equipment.

Small Equals Large — Small changes in physical activity and eating habits will, over time, make a huge difference.

Show Up — As Nike said, "Just Do It." Succeeding means doing it even when we'd rather not. Then, pretty soon, it becomes a habit.

LET ME HEAR FROM YOU

If you're taking the time to read the last few pages there's a pretty good chance that you liked the contents. Or, you could be like a professor I called on years ago, when I was selling college textbooks. I asked how he liked a book I was hoping he would use in one of his classes. He said, "Harry, I like the table of contents and the index, it's just all of the crap in between."

Many of the stories in this book were spontaneous responses to various chapters I sent to friends for review. They're some of the best stories in the book. If you have a story to tell, please send it to me

My website is **www.fitnessbeyondfifty.com**, email **Harry@fitnessbeyondfifty. com**. I plan to post stories on the website as well as information on fitness and health that hopefully will be of interest to you and others. Lots of research is being done in this field and much of it provides us with new insights that can be educational and motivational.

PLEASE TELL YOUR FRIENDS

If you like my book I hope you'll share that view with your friends. The success of a book like mine benefits enormously from word-of-mouth marketing. Someone will read it, like it and decide that it's useful information for their friends and relatives who need some education and motivation to get in shape. Some of those readers will read it, take action and share it with others. Ordering it is easy — just go to my website, listed above, or you can order from Amazon, Barnes and Noble or Google Books. Who knows, maybe it will go "viral," my new favorite word.

My motivation for writing this book was to encourage others to live a more active, healthy life. I plan to donate at least twenty percent of any earnings to health-related charities. I gain a lot of pleasure out of helping others. I hope I've helped you.

ABOUT THE AUTHOR

Harry H. Gaines is a retired publishing executive who's spent most of his adult life working to stay fit and eat healthy. Over the years his athletic activities have included running, swimming, tennis, golf, strength training and cycling. Today, in his early seventies, he's an active cyclist, logging 5,000 miles per year, plus active in strength training and golf. His wife, Debra A. Carrier, is also an active exerciser.

ACKNOWLEDGMENTS

In the spring of 2010, I met Scott Pullen of dotFIT, an online fitness and nutrition company, and he asked me to write some articles for his company's blog. While the articles I produced were decidedly mediocre, in my retrospective view, they got me started. Cathy Moschetto, director of our fitness center in SW Florida, read my articles and asked me to write some stories for her newsletter about what some members and staff have done to improve their fitness and health.

I sent some of the articles to several friends, including Pat Hedley, who repeatedly urged me to write a book on fitness and health. After about a month of her prodding I decided to give it a try. I was only seventy-two; why not take on something hard? Thanks, Pat; it wouldn't have happened without your encouragement. Your critique of the writing and the stories you've contributed were also outstanding.

Art Wester, my friend for over forty years, was initially the sole critic. I'd write something and send it to him for comments. Then I'd rewrite it and send it again. There's no question that his feedback had a major impact on the quality of this book. I wouldn't have gotten beyond the first chapter without his help.

When Bill Young, a CPA, and Halyna Traversa, a former general counsel, came to visit us in Bucks County, PA, I noticed her groaning aloud at grammatical errors as she read *The New York Times*. That's all I needed to know to recruit her and she's been terrific, much more than just a grammarian. Her husband Bill is also terrific, and they've both added excellent stories.

The number of reviewers just grew and grew, eventually reaching over twenty. Many read chapters multiple times. Art Kramer, Ph.D., Director of the Beckman Institute at the University of Illinois, is one of the top researchers in the area of exercise and the brain; he focused on his specific area of interest. Art's positive review was a real boost to my confidence.

Theodore L. Brown, Ph.D., an outstanding author in his own right, helped keep me out of trouble in the science topics, wrote great critical comments and suggested the final title. Roger Kelton, a PH.D. in exercise physiology who's also very knowledgeable about exercise kinesiology, was terrific in his science feedback but also in many other ways — and he didn't even know me. We met toward the end of the process.

Following are the additional reviewers who've been great critics and also provided excellent stories:

Chris Aland, M.D., John Allison, Margarita Bailey, Vicki Burton, Marvin Cashman, Bill Easton, Paul Feyen, Ann Fitzgibbons, Kathy Granger, Sandy Hackney, Bill Hollister, Judy Keenan, Betty Martin, Cathy Moschetto, David Nelson, M.D., David Ostrow, P.T., George Owens, Maureen Pease, D.V.M., Bill Pritts, Neale Sweet and David Walls.

When the manuscript was almost finished I corralled another group of friends to give it a look. Many provided excellent comments plus wrote stories that have added significantly to the quality of the book. They are: Ruth Barks, Tom Barry, Russ Campion, Len Carlson, Mary Anne Dignan, Sue Drosdzal, Harry Groth, Ron Larson, Marika Hartman, Tom Moe, Caroline Nielsen, Peggy Post, Alan Sachs, Bob Seidell, Sally Snyder, Mike Tiberi, D.D.S., Mark Tonnesen, Kathleen Wilson, M.D. and Tom Wilson. My copy editor, Elizabeth IlgenFritz, has not only done an outstanding job but has been great fun to work with.

My wife, Debra Carrier, has suffered through countless conversations during the development and has been a superb sounding board. She also prodded me into working harder on a title, which ultimately led to the final one suggested by Ted Brown.

The final product is very different and of higher quality than the one I initially envisioned due directly to the feedback and stories from my cadre of critics. Thanks, guys. You've made the process an adventure versus a job. I hope we've all had fun as well as learned a lot. It's encouraging that many of you have upped the ante of exercise as a direct result of reading my manuscript. I have, too.

APPENDIX

GOAL SETTING TEMPLATE

	Goal	Current	12 Mo Goal	1 Mo	2 Mo	3 Mo	4 Mo	5 Mo	6 Mo	7 Mo	8 Mo	9 Mo	10 Mo	11 Mo	12 Mo
Physical Goals	Weight														
	Waist Size														
	Blood Pressure														
Exercise Goals (10 Reps)	Chest Press														
	Upright Row														
	Bicep Curl														
	Leg Press														
Aerobics	Cycling – Dist/Avg Spd														
	Running – Dist/Avg Spd														
	Swimming – Laps														
	Walking – Dist/Avg Spd														
Check @ 6 Months	Cholesterol														
	HDL														
	LDL														
	Total														
	Triglycerides														
	Body Fat Percent														
	Glucose														

STRENGTH TRAINING EXERCISES

	Weight	Sets	Reps	Date	Date	Date	Date	Date	Date	Date	Date	Date	Date	Date	Date
Upper Body																
Bench Press																
Upright Row																
Bent Row																
Biceps Curl																
Triceps Extension																
Dumbbell Fly																
Pull Ups																
Push Ups																
Lower Body																
Squats																
Toe Raise																
Leg Press																
Leg Curl																
Leg Extension																
Core																
Abdominal Crunches																
Back Extensions																
Sitting or Incline Rotations																
Side Curl-Up, Fitball																

BOOKS AND WEBSITES

Tom Hanks played the part of an attorney in the movie, "Philadelphia." He told this story: Question: "What do you have when you have 200 lawyers at the bottom of the ocean? Answer: A good start."

Reading this book represents a good start. It'll help if you read more plus check out websites that can provide you with information in a timely manner. They'll keep you going when you may not be in the mood.

Following are some that I found helpful in the writing of this book as well as in providing me with inspiration and education over the years. This is in no way a definitive list. I did make a list of all of the articles, books and other sources I utilized. It ran to over fifteen pages, which I decided was way more than anyone would want to know.

NEWSLETTERS AND WEBSITES

Active.com — There are many writers for this website; the fitness and health topics covered are presented in a clear, simple manner. Signing up is free.

Choosemyplate.gov — Prepared by the USDA, it has the latest recommendations for healthy eating. The site is loaded with useful information for all age groups. I highly recommend it.

Drmirkin.com — Gabe Mirkin, in his seventies, writes a weekly column on a wide range of health and exercise topics. He's a retired M.D. who's been an active athlete all of his life. He and his wife ride their tandem bicycle nearly every day and still compete in some races. You can sign up for his free newsletter plus order a free copy of his ebook on the next page. It's excellent information.

Mayoclinic.com — It's hard to find a better website; almost anything you want to know about exercise and diet can be found here. You can access one of my favorites by typing "Slide Show: Weight Training Exercises" in the search section. It lists a variety of exercises and provides step-by-step directions on how to do them.

Mytpi.com — This provides access to the Titleist Performance Institute, which is useful for a variety of sports, not just golf. Dr. Greg Rose and Dave Phillips describe various exercises and offer a step-by-step summary that you can print as well as a video showing the steps. You can also print the pictures to be sure you remember how to do the exercises properly.

Realage.com — You can fill out a questionnaire to determine your "real age" based on your exercise and eating habits. They'll also provide regular updates of information.

BOOKS

Exercise

Bring It! By Tony Horton, 2011, Rodale — A book with excellent illustrations and step-by-step exercise procedures as well as fitness plans. Horton is the creator of the P90X program.

Core Performance by Mark Verstegen, 2004, Rodale — It has exercises for core and overall strength training with excellent pictures. This is one of my favorites.

The Life Plan by Jeffrey S. Life, M.D., Ph.D., 2011, Atria Books — A new book written by an M.D. who got the exercise religion in his early sixties. Lots of "how-to" information.

Dr. Gabe Mirkin's Pocket Guide to Fitness and Sports, by Gabe Mirkin, 1998 — About sixty pages, available online free as an ebook when you sign up for Gabe's weekly newsletter.

Serious Training for Endurance Athletes, 2nd edition, 1996, by Sleamaker and Browning, Human Kinetics — While this is considered a must-read for serious athletes, it's also helpful to all of us. I've used it as a valuable reference since the first edition was published in 1989.

Strength Training Anatomy by Frederic Delavier, 2006, Human Kinetics — A must-have, in my view. It shows the anatomy and names for muscle groups plus how to execute various exercises. The illustrations are beautiful.

Stretching — All of the stretching books listed have very good to excellent illustrations.

Stretching Anatomy by Nelson and Kokkonen, 2007, Human Kinetics (my favorite).

The Stark Reality of Stretching by Dr. Steven D. Stark, 1997, Stark Reality Corp.

Stretching by Anderson, 2010, Shelter Publications — Over three and a half million copies sold since 1980. The illustrations leave something to be desired in comparison to newer books but still a classic.

Exercise and the Brain

Spark: The Revolutionary New Science of Exercise and the Brain by Ratey and Hagerman, 2008, Little Brown — The Naperville School District story in the first chapter is fascinating. Chapter Two, "Learning: Grow Your Brain Cells" and Chapter Nine, "Aging: The Wise Way" are my favorites.

Willpower: Rediscovering The Greatest Human Strength by Baumeister and Tierney, 2011, Penguin Press — Well-written, interesting and educational; all of the features I like in a good book.

Healthy Eating

The Mayo Clinic Diet: Eat Well. Enjoy Life. Lose Weight by the Mayo Clinic staff, 2010, Good Books — Well-written, beautifully illustrated, practical suggestions; a winner.

The Spectrum: A Scientifically Proven Program to Feel Better, Live Longer, Lose Weight, Gain Health by Dean Ornish, M.D., 2007, Ballantine Books — I confess to not having read it but my wife thinks it's terrific, as does my friend Art Wester.

Omnivore's Dilemma by Michael Pollan, 2006, Penguin Books — Pollan is a good and thoughtful writer.

INDEX